Richard W. Roukema, MD

The Soul in Distress
What Every Pastoral Counselor Should Know About Emotional and Mental Illness

Pre-publication
REVIEW

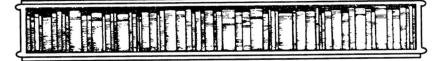

The Soul in Distress
What Every Pastoral Counselor Should Know About Emotional and Mental Illness

THE HAWORTH PRESS
New, Recent, and Forthcoming Titles
of Related Interest

Growing Up: Pastoral Nurture for the Later Years by Thomas B. Robb

Religion and the Family: When God Helps by Laurel Arthur Burton

Victims of Dementia: Services, Support, and Care by Wm. Michael Clemmer

Horrific Traumata: A Pastoral Response to the Post-Traumatic Stress Disorder by N. Duncan Sinclair

Aging and God: Spiritual Pathways to Mental Health in Midlife and Later Years by Harold G. Koenig

Counseling for Spiritually Empowered Wholeness: A Hope-Centered Approach by Howard Clinebell

Shame: A Faith Perspective by Robert H. Albers

Dealing with Depression: Five Pastoral Interventions by Richard Dayringer

Righteous Religion: Unmasking the Illusions of Fundamentalism and Authoritarian Catholicism by Kathleen Y. Ritter and Craig W. O'Neill

Theological Context for Pastoral Caregiving: Word in Deed by Howard Stone

Pastoral Care in Pregnancy Loss: A Ministry Long Needed by Thomas Moe

A Gospel for the Mature Years: Finding Fulfillment by Knowing and Using Your Gifts by Harold Koenig, Tracy Lamar, and Betty Lamar

Is Religion Good for Your Health? The Effects of Religion on Physical and Mental Health by Harold Koenig

The Soul in Distress: What Every Pastoral Counselor Should Know About Emotional and Mental Illness by Richard Roukema

The Soul in Distress
What Every Pastoral Counselor Should Know About Emotional and Mental Illness

Richard W. Roukema, MD

The Haworth Pastoral Press
An Imprint of The Haworth Press, Inc.
New York • London

4/01

Published by

The Haworth Pastoral Press, an imprint of The Haworth Press, Inc., 10 Alice Street, Binghamton, NY 13904-1580

Cover design by Monica L. Seifert.

Library of Congress Cataloging-in-Publication Data

Roukema, Richard W.
The soul in distress: what every pastoral counselor should know about emotional and mental illness / Richard W. Roukema.
Xiii, 274 p. cm.   Bib. p. 253-257
Includes bibliographical references and index.
ISBN 0-7890-0168-3 (alk. paper).
1. Mentally ill–Pastoral counseling of. 2. Mental illness.
I. Title.
BV4461.R68 1997
259′42–dc21

96-48818
CIP

To Todd Richard Roukema
1959-1976

A loving and courageous spirit
May peace and tranquility be his just reward

ABOUT THE AUTHOR

Richard W. Roukema, MD, FAPA, is Clinical Associate Professor of Psychiatry at the University of Medicine and Dentistry of New Jersey and a psychiatrist in private practice in Ridgewood. He was trained in psychiatry at Columbia University, College of Physicians and Surgeons, and is a graduate of the W. A. White Institute of Psychoanalysis. As Associate Director of the University Hospital Psychiatric Center, he lectured to medical students, psychiatry residents, nurses, and physicians and was the recipient of several teaching awards. Currently Director of Continuing Medical Education and Director of Outpatient Mental Health Services at the Ramapo Ridge Psychiatric Hospital, Dr. Roukema is a member of the American Psychiatric Association and the American Medical Association. He appeared on WABC New York's half-hour documentary on teenage suicide called "I'd Rather Be Dead." He is married to Republican Congresswoman Marge Roukema of New Jersey. They have two married children, Meg and Greg.

CONTENTS

Foreword

This is a book of explanation. Dr. Richard Roukema has given us a carefully crafted book that explains issues of psychiatry and pastoral counseling, which the clergyperson needs to know if he or she is going to have an informed ministry.

This book gives excellent background information for the concerned pastoral caregiver. It examines the genetic and biochemical understanding of mental illness and the effects of parenting, heredity, and society. Then, after providing us a background through which to look, Dr. Roukema clarifies the differences between the more specific clinical disorders and what a pastoral counselor will encounter dealing with people suffering in these ways. There is clarity and important insights concerning how to deal with and help people suffering from such disorders. The pastor is called upon to respond differently to a person who is depressed than to a person who is paranoid or narcissistic. Some people need comfort; others need confrontation. Some need to be included in many parts of the life of an active congregation; others need thoughtful exclusion from activities that would not be helpful to them or others.

The strength of this book, from my perspective, is its understanding of how people suffering from different types of emotional problems impact a congregation and a pastor, and how the bewildering traps and pain that are inflicted can be avoided or turned into successful intervention or circumvented disaster. This can happen only if we are educated and prepared. It is important for the congregational leader to understand the pitfalls into which he or she can easily fall. It is critical to see the pain and to know how to reach out with caring or how to confront directly the kind of person who will easily undermine a religious community and a ministry.

When I read Dr. Roukema's chapter "Personality Disorders," I wrote to him, "It couldn't be better. Clear, concise, good sense of meaning. . . . The idea of learning how to work with and survive the difficult parishioner rather than change him is important." After reading several other chapters, I wrote, "I am very impressed. . . . I think that your section on transference is particularly well written and valuable." That has been my reaction throughout.

This is a very specialized book for the religious leader who wants to have a resource with clear information about people who populate every congregation. If we look into ourselves, we can see pieces of these descriptions and can understand the pain and the distortions that come with this suffering. We can also understand how we should react to people who present themselves to us in these ways and be more able to create the environment that will allow for a healthy interaction.

I highly recommend this book.

James C. Wyrtzen, DMin
The Blanton-Peale Graduate Institute

Acknowledgments

A very special thanks to Reverend James Wyrtzen, who faithfully read each chapter, made invaluable suggestions, and encouraged me to continue during the early phases of this book. Much appreciation to Reverend Douglas Fromm, my pastor, who gave me ideas and inspiration during our lunches together. To other members of the clergy who have nourished and sustained me and my family throughout the years, I am grateful.

I am indebted to Drs. William Layman, Steven Simring, Richard Frances, and Sheldon Miller for their time and encouragement.

It was a pleasure to work with the editors from The Haworth Press: Bill Palmer, Susan Gibson, Peg Marr, and Lisa Franko, all most courteous and professional.

My agent, Maryanne Colas, was an enormous help in the early review of chapters. Her persistent enthusiasm and cheerleading helped me through the long hours. To Eileen Flynn, an accomplished author, I owe a special thanks because of her careful review of the manuscript when it was in raw form. Thanks to Diane Fallon for her suggestions. I also wish to acknowledge the secretarial help of Judy Van Dyke and Linda Davis, who were always available to do the basic work behind the scene.

To my wife, Marge, my daughter, Meg, and son, Greg, I owe a loving hug for all their encouragement to my writing. God's grace.

Chapter 1

Introduction: Conflicts and Concerns of Religion and Psychiatry

Recently I had lunch with a close friend who is the pastor of a local church. He told me that there are some members of his church who are very difficult to understand. He said:

> I have a man in my church who seems to get everyone riled up. He has a way of polarizing people. He manages to split people into groups and is very disruptive. He's very impulsive, and people either love him or hate him. It makes some of my congregants want to quit the group. And he drives me crazy.

At the time we discussed this, it seemed to me that the pastor was dealing with a situation that is not too unusual in congregations. Every psychiatrist would recognize the potential here for huge problems for any clergyperson. In all probability, he was dealing with a congregant who had a borderline personality. When I further described the characteristics of this disorder, my friend had the look of recognition on his face.

This conversation moved me to consider the clergyperson's dilemma. He or she must relate to a large group of people in a variety of situations and adapt to each congregant's peculiar ways. At the same time, he or she must aspire to be a paragon of virtue, always behaving in an idealized and perhaps restricted manner. While meeting the emotional needs of the congregation, the clergyperson also has to be there to give inspiration every week, even if he or she does not feel very inspired at that moment.

To be at funerals one day, weddings the next day; to serve as administrator, friend, counselor, husband, father, wife, mother, and

1

role model all at the same time–this has to be one of the most demanding jobs that I can imagine. It is good that the clergyperson has God on his or her side!

As a psychiatrist, I deal with patients on a close, personal basis, usually one at a time, rather than in groups. I believe that I have a much easier time of it than my clergyman friend. Furthermore, I have the advantage of extensive training in the area of understanding the human condition from the psychological viewpoint, to which the clergy has little exposure unless they are involved in the field of pastoral counseling.

Most clergy, however, do not have special training in pastoral counseling. It is my conviction that these clergypersons or any pastoral caregiver could benefit from insights that have been uncovered in the field of psychiatry. He or she could profit from reading a psychiatrist's comments about the emotions and behavior of patients and reflections on counseling them. There are always new discoveries in psychiatry: new brain scans, psychotropic drugs, new ways to handle emotional problems. I believe that some familiarity with these areas are necessary for today's clergy.

Since pastoral caregivers are constantly dealing with distressed congregants, the information in this book will assist them in making their work less difficult and more rewarding. While attempting to be helpful, the book does not purport to be a short course in pastoral counseling. To be an expert in this field, it requires many hours of training, supervision, and personal analysis.

A LOOK BACKWARD

Some years ago, when I first entered the field of psychiatry, there was considerable fear among religious people about psychiatry and psychoanalysis in particular. This fear, especially among very conservative groups, remains to some extent even today.

Some individuals regarded psychiatry as an atheistic philosophy or an evil that had to be avoided or even attacked. The fundamentalist religions, as well as Catholicism, were originally rather hostile to the notion that a series of mental constructions such as Freud had proclaimed, based on sex and aggression, could possibly be of any help to people who were religious. Besides, Freud appeared to be an atheist or, at best, an agnostic. He declared in his writings that religion was merely a wish or an illusion to meet the insecurity of those who were troubled. As Erich Fromm states in his book *Sigmund Freud's Mission*,

> [Freud] made his attitude very explicit [about religion] in various writings, especially in the *Future of an Illusion*. He sees in the belief in God a fixation to the longing for an all-protecting father figure, an expression of a wish to be helped and saved, when in reality man can, if not save himself, at least help himself, only by waking up from childish illusions and by using his own strength, his reason and skills. (p. 95)

Many patients who I have counseled in the past, who came from religious backgrounds, were frankly frightened by the teachings of Freud. As a result, many of these troubled persons sought help for their problems from the clergy, often with considerable success, and sometimes with obvious failures–depending on the nature of the problem.

As the years have gone by, there has been a definite easing of tension between the clergy and the field of psychiatry, and an active cooperation has occurred. However, conservative religious people still fear "atheistic" psychiatry. The fear of these groups is not without some foundation. Some psychiatrists have been openly hostile toward religion. Most have ignored its importance, and others have smiled benignly at the mention of spiritual and religious beliefs. I think it is safe to say that most psychiatrists do not inquire about their patient's religious concerns. Yet, in the minds of some patients, their faith represents the most powerful force they can possess for living effectively.

Back in the 1940s, Dr. Smiley Blanton, a psychoanalyst in New York City, and Dr. Norman Vincent Peale, pastor of the Marble Collegiate Church and author of *The Power of Positive Thinking*, founded a clinic in New York City dedicated to the collaboration of psychiatrists and clergy for the purpose of offering the best help to those who are troubled. The clinic and training program is known as The Institute of Religion and Health. In addition to treating many emotionally disturbed individuals, the institute trains clergypersons to become competent pastoral counselors.

While such a clinic successfully melds the concerns of the emotionally upset religious person, most psychotherapists practicing in this country neglect the importance of religion in the patient's life. It would be helpful if psychotherapists took the time to understand the nature of religious experience and the degree to which religion can assist the psychotherapeutic process. Although the clergy has become much more informed about the psychological issues troubling their congregants, psychotherapists have failed to appreciate the impact of religious forces in the lives of their patients.

I believe that most of the clergy are very aware of the close relationship between the religious and emotional experiences of their congregants. For example, mood disturbances can greatly affect one's thoughts about religion. Some people are religious only when they become depressed. By contrast, others find it difficult to address God when struggling with depression. Some people are religious only when anxious or distressed; others only during a time of significant loss. It seems to me, therefore, that the clergy should become as informed as possible about the latest findings in the field of mental health. By doing so, the clergy can optimize their effectiveness in working with congregants who are emotionally distraught.

In recent years, the advances in the field of psychiatry have been enormous. We know more about how the mind functions; we know more about how the brain operates and what interferes with brain metabolism. While the clergy have felt increasingly at ease and have worked cooperatively with psychiatrists and other psychotherapists, it has been very difficult for the clergy to keep up with the important new discoveries in the treatment of the emotionally and mentally ill. I am certain that psychiatrists have not kept abreast of changes in religious developments, either. Only recently has there been some discussion in psychiatric journals by psychiatrists such as David Larson and others about the effect of religion on the emotional life of patients.

Before describing the general field of psychiatry, it would be beneficial to understand the common areas of concern that the clergy and psychiatrists share.

COMMON ROLES

The clergy and psychiatrists have much in common. At times they perform similar functions and use similar methods. Both hear about the painful experiences that people encounter.

Ventilation has been considered by both groups as essential to beginning any kind of counseling. Ventilation has, of course, many benefits. By sharing emotional conflicts with an interested and empathic listener, one can feel considerable relief from anxiety. Furthermore, in ventilating, the individual's problems often become clearer merely by speaking about or formulating them.

One day, while listening intently to a patient ventilate, it occurred to me, with apologies to Alexander Pope, that "to ventilate is human, to be listened to, divine." I am certain that most of us have had the experience of being very comforted through the process of ventilation, especially when dealing with an overwhelming problem.

By ventilating, the person verbalizes his or her feelings, thoughts, and views. The therapist/counselor, meanwhile, listens for an underlying problem or attitude about which the person is only dimly aware, and asks leading questions and elicits the more basic problems that exist. He or she then is better able to formulate the nature of the distraught person's difficulties.

Ventilation often involves confession, particularly in the consulting room of the clergy. In the Roman Catholic Church, confession has historically been formalized, although there has been far less stress on confession recently. Confession in other religious groups has been practiced with or without an intervening priest or clergyman.

Revealing perceived misdeeds (sins) has always been comforting to the sinner. In many religions, confession is followed by absolution of guilt and reconciliation with a Higher Being. As a result, confession often contributes to equanimity and to a feeling of oneness with the world and with one's Higher Being.

Confession in the setting of psychotherapy has been regarded by many as an important ingredient in the therapeutic crucible. However, confession in psychotherapy can be misused. It is not uncommon for an individual who has committed adultery to go to a psychotherapist to tell all, rather than to a clergyman. Sometimes, in fact, therapy is used as implied permission to continue with the perceived wrongdoing. When a therapist, in the attempt to be neutral and not condemning, has neither condoned the action nor forbidden it, the patient sometimes interprets this as permission to continue to do as he or she pleases.

Confession can also be compulsive in nature and become in itself neurotic. By bringing every felt misdeed into the therapy session, the person hopes to absolve him or herself of guilt. Often, this process continues without the patient being consciously aware of it. The therapist may perceive this as a repetitive "dumping" of the guilt on his or her lap. This pattern needs to be corrected to ensure that therapy is not misused. Particularly among obsessive-compulsive people, there is a tendency to use confession in this manner.

In the counseling done by both clergy and psychiatrists, emotional excesses are frequently encountered. Anger, fear, resentment, depression, anxiety, and panic are very common. It should be noted here that some extremes of emotion are not merely psychological events or the result of psychological problems. Often such symptoms are produced primarily by biological disturbances. This occurs, for example, in manic-depressive disorder, which will be discussed in Chapter 4, "Mood Disorders: Depression and Manic States." The clergy should be aware that not all emotional extremes are due to external stress. Many physical diseases also cause nervous symptoms. This will be discussed in some detail in considering organic mental disorders.

After the patient/congregant expresses extremes in emotion, the clergyperson or the psychotherapist can probe beneath the surface to uncover the sources of these disturbances. Having a trusted person with whom to discuss one's fears and anxieties is a great relief to those who avail themselves of such a relationship. Clarifying underlying problems and working on solutions can be very gratifying to both the counselor and the counseled. Some emotional problems take considerable time to work through, and it requires patience and persistence to solve the more difficult dilemmas that confront disturbed individuals. In addition to psychotherapy, where indicated, the psychiatrist can use medications or other physical modalities for treatment of major psychiatric illnesses.

HISTORICAL CHANGES

An interesting change has occurred historically in the views of organized religion toward mental illness. Very few religious groups, now, do not accept epilepsy as a genuine disease, whereas in the past, it had been associated with devil possession or some mental derangement allegedly due to evil forces. Similarly, persons who are now diagnosed as schizophrenic often were regarded in the past as either saints or sinners. Today, most people in the Western world consider schizophrenia to be a mental illness.

The notion of faith healing has been explored by clergy and physicians alike. The question remains unanswered as to how extensively one's prayers can affect physical disease. There are cases on record in the medical world that show spontaneous cures even with the worst diseases, such as inoperable cancer. There are no immediate explanations for these. If these cures happen to be associated with the prayers of the fervent believer, then the cures, of course, are ascribed to faith healing (that is, to miracles). Many of these cases, however, involve people who have made no claims to faith in a God or any use of prayer for healing.

It has been my observation that if a patient has a deep religious faith, he or she usually contends with physical disease much better than without such faith. Of course, there are exceptions to this as well. It is tragic when someone continues to deteriorate with a serious disease, such as cancer, and then ascribes this to the fact that he or she does not have enough faith. I have seen this happen in several instances.

Recently, there has been much interest in the attitude and state of mind of a person suffering from a major illness. Norman Cousins has written books for the layperson on this subject. One of them is *Head First*. In it, he gives many examples of how positive attitudes affected the course of illness, not necessarily curing the disease, but at least enabling the individual so afflicted to deal with illness in a more positive manner.

Furthermore, it has been demonstrated that the immune system is adversely affected by clinical depression, an effect that is greater with advancing age. This implies that the person with clinical depression is less protected by the immune system than when he or she is free of depression. The phenomenon reverses itself when the depression is gone. This work was done by Drs. Stephen Schleifer and Steven Keller of the University of New Jersey, Departments of Medicine, Psychiatry, and Dentistry, and Marvin Stein at the Mount Sinai School of Medicine, City University of New York.

Much more research must be done to specifically establish the importance of stress and psychological factors on the course of physical and mental illness. But while such research proceeds, there is little doubt that the spiritual aspect of any patient's life needs more attention from both the clergy and the psychotherapist.

WHAT PSYCHIATRY CAN DO

Although there are many common areas of concern in the counseling served by the clergy and psychiatrists, there are also situations in which a knowledge of psychiatry would be extremely helpful to the clergy in enabling them to refer clients properly. Even a rudimentary knowledge of psychiatry can help the clergy facilitate their care of congregants who are distressed.

The first example illustrates how an organic illness can masquerade as an emotional problem of psychological origin. The second example shows how religious guilt can arise from a psychotic process associated with depression.

Case 1: Bill

One day, I saw a 50-year-old man named Bill in the emergency room of the local hospital. Bill was very disturbed, with paranoid thoughts and agitation. Anyone could recognize that he was psychotic. I had never seen him before, but I learned that he was in therapy with a nonmedical psychotherapist for problems regarding his daughter and her husband. There were long-standing difficulties with this relationship. The problems mostly concerned the father's inability to accept his son-in-law.

While in the process of discussing these problems with his psychotherapist on the day of admission to the hospital, the patient had suddenly developed extreme, erratic behavior, which was totally out of character for him; he became grossly psychotic. The therapist's interpretation of this behavior was that the father could not accept his daughter's marriage, and that he felt extremely competitive with his son-in-law, presumably because of the father's close attachment to his daughter.

Although the patient developed grossly psychotic behavior, the therapist insisted on viewing this as a totally psychological problem. While it is true that some psychotic behaviors appear to be reactive phenomena, it is a mistake to assume that all psychotic behavior is the result of emotional problems. Most psychotic disorders are primarily due to organic or biological abnormalities, as will be discussed later.

Bill was admitted to the hospital and placed on the psychiatric unit because of his extreme symptoms. He had disrobed himself and was standing naked on his bed; he was completely out of contact with reality. His blood pressure on admission was 220 over 120, which represented a severe hypertensive reaction. Bill was treated medically for the high blood pressure and, within five days, he returned to normal. His behavior was much the same as it had been prior to his hospitalization.

The patient was diagnosed as having hypertensive encephalopathy. This condition can occur with or without stress and can manifest itself as either severely increased blood pressure with headaches, or, as it did in this case, as a severe psychosis.

Meanwhile, the psychotherapist who had been treating the patient continued to insist that the psychosis was purely the result of the psychological problem; he did not recognize the existence of the physical illness as a possible etiological factor. Underlying this assumption is the notion that all abnormal behavior is the result of emotional problems. It also assumes that when one event precedes the other, the first event is the cause of the second—a common logical fallacy.

I monitored Bill at my office for over a year, and he did not have a recurrence of the hypertension. His family problem, however, did not resolve quickly. After time, he did seem to develop a somewhat better relationship with his family. At the very least, if things were not fully resolved, they were certainly more quiescent.

It is unclear why a hypertensive crisis occurs. As a rule, it is not a simple psychologically based phenomenon. There are many biological factors at work that one must recognize. The condition cannot be treated merely by psychological means. As in this example, it is important to consider that organic disease can cause marked changes in behavior. Thus, when treating psychological and behavioral changes, it is important to remember that there are both emotional and physical causes of illness. Another example of the overlap in organic and psychological factors is the following.

Case 2: Nell

Nell, a middle-aged woman, gradually developed severe depression, lost considerable weight, and reported that she had "sinned against the Holy Spirit." She felt that she could not be forgiven and feared that she had caused tragedies in the lives of other persons merely by having had bad thoughts about them.

In dealing with such a phenomenon, an inexperienced clergyperson might attempt to try to resolve the patient's problem by dealing with the issue of guilt. With every good intention, he or she might try to reassure the congregant that such guilt is unwarranted and recommend prayer in order to overcome the problem.

This case history illustrates a symptom frequently seen by psychiatrists in patients who are depressed. It represents evidence of delusional thinking (i.e., irrational beliefs inconsistent with the patient's background or culture). People who are clinically depressed have low self-esteem, self-deprecatory ideas, and at times, delusions (delusional depression).

In this condition, the individual feels that he or she is evil and may even feel possessed by the devil. Frequently, the religious person says, "I have sinned against the Holy Spirit," which among orthodox Christians represents the ultimate defiance of God, the "unforgivable sin." Any attempt to treat this delusional thinking by purely psychological means is doomed to failure. Such thoughts, occurring during a depression, are distortions in the patient's normal thought patterns. Although these thoughts are related to the patient's life and religious background, these ideas should not be dealt with as a current reality. Rather, if the patient is treated with appropriate antipsychotic and antidepressant medications, the symptoms usually resolve within a few weeks. Gradually, the patient is no longer distressed by irrational ideas, and her thoughts return to normal. Following this, any residual guilt–actual or neurotic–can be dealt with in therapy in a rational way.

These two examples are presented to demonstrate the combination of psychological and organic factors that must be considered to successfully help the patient. It is important to differentiate between illnesses that can be handled by expert counseling and other ailments that require active psychiatric and medical intervention.

The purpose of this book is to highlight the latest findings in the field of psychiatry in order to inform the clergy of different treatment methods for the emotionally and mentally ill. A number of practical suggestions will also be offered in order to assist the clergyperson in the often difficult work with congregants.

It will become clear that these suggestions and treatment modalities complement the work of the clergy without in any way conflicting with theology. It is my contention that the conflict between psychotherapists and the clergy, where it exists, is the result of personal attitudes on the part of some psychotherapists who, in their efforts to be scientific or noncommittal in a religious sense, scare off those who place a high priority on faith and religion. In addition, there are some psychotherapists who are clearly hostile to religion or are so humanistic in their attitudes that they frighten the more spiritually sensitive. My impression is that there are many psychotherapists who ignore the religious attitudes of their patients because of their own lack of familiarity or comfort with religion. I think there is a need for religious training for psychotherapists as well as psychological training for theologians.

Psychology involves the emotions and the intellect; it can never be separated completely from matters of faith and the existential concerns of the soul. As the seventeenth-century physician/theologian Pascal said, "The heart has its reasons which reason knows nothing of." Matters of faith are very important to many people. Such concerns should be considered important by psychotherapists. This does not mean that the lay counselor should advise the counseled in matters of the soul. There is plenty of work for everyone. The

clergyperson is needed in the spiritual domain and the psychotherapist in the psychological and emotional areas. Of course, the two
roles overlap, and every attempt ought to be made to understand the
contribution of the other. There is a need for the healthy interchange
of ideas between the two groups, a need which has not been met
very well in our society.

Chapter 2

Parents, Society, and Heredity

It happened about 25 years ago. I walked into a middle-class home to talk to a distressed father. His son had just run away from home, and he was trying to determine what he should do. We discussed the possibilities of his son's whereabouts and what to do next: call the police, wait for him to call home, or call his friends.

I reflected on the emotional and psychological reasons for the youngster's leaving home. The father heard my explanations but was not buying into my psychiatric reasoning. He indulged me for a while and then said with conviction, "It's all in the genes. That kid is just like his uncle, and there is nothing that we can do about it."

My psychiatric knowledge, at that point in time, told me that this misinformed father just did not understand the situation. How could he blame his son's aberrant behavior on family background, on heredity? Everybody in my field knew that improper mothering and fathering caused poor behavior later on in a child's life. We even knew that cold, withdrawn mothers caused schizophrenia. It was a classic case of denial on the part of the father. What ignorance! How could he not know that the improper parenting of his son had caused him to run away? So went my thoughts.

Many years have gone by, and we have learned some things that temper those rigid views. The father was partly right; but, he also had some things to learn about fathering. In the time that has elapsed, many changes have occurred in society that have influenced childrearing and behavior. In addition, important insights about heredity have been discovered through research. In this chapter as well as in the chapter on personality disorders, the role that parents play, the impact of culture on childrearing, and the new research on heredity will be elaborated in some detail.

Background

Prior to the psychoanalytic movement at the turn of the century, it was generally assumed that hereditary factors played a significant part in the formation of character, behavior, mannerisms, and—of course—appearance. Bloodlines are and were important to everyone.

Even today, every grandparent sees in his or her grandchildren the family resemblances in terms of physiognomy and traits such as stubbornness, creativity, intelligence, and craftsmanship. "He's just like his Uncle Bill," "She's as stubborn as her Aunt Jane," and "He's a chip off the old block" are common observations.

THE FREUDIAN REVOLUTION:
THE SHIFT TO PARENTAL RESPONSIBILITY

Having acknowledged such truisms as basic and infallible, people were shocked to learn of Freud's assertions regarding childrearing. Here was a neurologist from Vienna who invented a method of treatment he called "psychoanalysis." This method was based on his claim that the origin of "neurosis," as he called it, was due to conflicts resulting from improper childrearing. Freud maintained that faulty parental management of a child's sexual and aggressive impulses resulted in neurotic behavior. Furthermore, Freud claimed that the neurotic symptoms could be modified or eliminated by utilizing the "talking cure." The symptoms of neurosis were the result of conflict between the id (unconscious) impulses and the superego (loosely defined as the conscience), while the ego (or self) was valiantly attempting to direct the internal energies toward a resolution of the given conflict. If one failed to repress the conflict and remove it to the unconscious, or if other defense mechanisms did not adequately handle the conflict, a neurosis ensued. Thus spoke Freud and his disciples.

EFFECT ON CHILDREARING

Psychoanalysts in Europe and America began to pontificate on the subject of childrearing. Books, magazines, and newspaper articles implied or stated bluntly that the emotional miseries that mankind suffered were exclusively the result of poor or inadequate childrearing.

Parental guilt reigned supreme. Even in the 1980s, parents assumed that all aberrant behavior of their children was the result of poor parenting. It had to be someone's *fault.* The belief has long been held that a child is born with a *tabula rasa* (a clean slate), on which the parents, with their parental skills or lack thereof, write the fate of the child before the latter has a chance to determine his or her own destiny.

Psychotherapists of all kinds began to be challenged by adult patients to answer the question in the manner of Sherlock Holmes: "Who did it?" "Who is responsible for my neurosis?" "Which parent is to blame?" The questions did not imply any individual responsibility, and the inquirers basked in the self-satisfaction of pinning the blame on others, especially parents. For some patients, long periods of psychoanalysis followed, and after finding the "villain," the person's neurosis was not necessarily altered. Perhaps more than at any other time, after Freud's theories gained a following, ensued a period when parents were blamed for poor childrearing, and most parents readily assumed that blame.

THE SHIFT TO SOCIAL CAUSES

During the 1960s and 1970s, we witnessed the age of the unrepressed child and adolescent. At this time, the influence of heredity was minimized to a fault. Youth rejected the historical perspective and proceeded to reinvent every basic assumption of the adult world. In this cauldron of activity, parents had less and less control. Society was contributing to the development of the child in strange and different ways, while parents looked helplessly on. Meanwhile, parents continued to ask the question. "What have we done wrong?"

There probably has never been any period in history that has seen such remarkable social, ethical, and institutional changes in such a short span of time. Regardless of a person's heredity and strong family life, the child of the 1960s had to be tremendously affected by the instability of this difficult age.

It was during these two decades that student rebellion was rampant, the drug culture became prominent, and the sexual revolution was born. Among the other changes were the emergence of an organized woman's liberation and the civil rights movements in the United States. Religious and political institutions were demythologized and authority figures of all kinds were criticized. Minority activism and egalitarianism became common. R.D. Laing, a psychiatrist in England, blamed society for mental illness; in America, Thomas Szasz maintained that mental illness did not exist but was a myth fostered by the psychiatric profession. There were marked changes in education with new emphasis on values clarification and declining interest in the importance of actual information. Things that were "old" were useless; only the "new" was revered.

From the wide sweep of cultural change came many changes in acceptable behavior. The pressure on the growing child to be independent, to use drugs, to experiment with sexuality, or to engage in antiauthoritarian behavior was immense. Sibling and peer pressures in adolescence began to rival the input of parents, whose influence diminished markedly as societal factors became more dominant and persuasive. This left many parents relatively powerless in the area of childrearing. Some blamed their children's problems on the rapid changes in society.

However, the prevailing climate did not make most parents feel less guilty. Many continued to be hounded by the conviction that parents always determined the fate of the child. If the child failed at school and did not become a responsible adult, parents inevitably assumed the blame. If the child did grow to maturity without significant problems, parents felt they were directly responsible for the child's success as well. Only recently have parents begun to place the blame on the schools their children attend or on television and other factors outside of the family.

REACTIONS TO SOCIAL CHANGES

When there are rapid changes in society, there are usually groups or institutions that arise to fill the void left by such alterations. People do not function well without some leadership. They look for new models.

The commune was an attempt to remake the family that had been rejected in adolescence, and the adoption of Eastern religions by the young was a search for spiritual fulfillment to substitute for the old religions that they had abandoned.

Many parents reacted to the social upheaval of the 1960s and 1970s by joining a group called Tough Love–a self-help group that teaches tough parenting to families that are falling apart. The group encourages setting very definite limits on childrearing, creating a united front on the part of the parents, and expressing strong, but positive reactions to aberrant behavior. Hopefully, this is done in the context of expressing love for the child and with his or her welfare in mind.

Individuals reacted to the social changes by joining groups such as EST (Erhardt Seminar Training) and Life Spring, which emphasized the role of individual responsibility for the person's success and happiness. In many ways, these groups resemble traditional religions in that the responsibility for one's life is placed squarely on the person. The basic message is "Don't blame others for your unhappiness. Only you can change things; no one will do it for you."

Thus, while parents were blaming themselves for being inadequate parents or blaming the deteriorating society, many of their offspring were trying to do what generations of children have typically done–build a better life based on values discovered through their own searching experience in the new groups that emerged.

But is all behavior determined only by the influence of parents and the surrounding culture within which a child grows? Although many people have long suspected that heredity also plays a large part in our behavior, researchers have only recently begun to study heredity in a systematic fashion.

In Chapter 10, "Personality Disorders," I discuss the different temperaments that children have at birth and how little these change when observed over a 20-year period. The mix of the infant's temperament with his or her parents' personalities and the influence of society all help to determine the adult personality.

But the specific effects of heredity on the individual have been studied mainly in patients with physical and mental disease, not in cases of normal development. In the following section, I will address the latest findings in the research on certain important mental illnesses.

RESEARCH ON HEREDITY OF MENTAL ILLNESS

Research in psychiatry has recently discovered some interesting findings in the heredity of some illnesses, especially in the serious psychoses. Although some of the neurotic disorders such as anxiety, phobias, obsessive-compulsive disorders, and psychosomatic disorders also show some hereditary transmission, they do so with much less frequency. Many mental illnesses have been found to have strong hereditary or biological causes. For example, schizophrenia was regarded as a parent-induced disease only 20 years ago. The psychiatric literature offered the "schizophrenogenic mother" and "refrigerator parents" to describe the origins of the illness. Examples were cited of poor parental communication with children and of the "double-bind" phenomenon, in which parents gave contradictory messages to their children, thus creating instability, insecurity, and possibly schizophrenia.

Modern research, including studies of heredity involving twins, has shown little evidence that the child's environment is the primary factor in producing schizophrenia. It has become evident that the causes of a major psychosis such as schizophrenia are multifactorial, and that much more research is necessary to discover just to what extent heredity is responsible for this illness.

The following facts about schizophrenia have been observed through research thus far:

1. For years, it has been shown that approximately 1 percent of newborns will develop schizophrenia some time in their lives.
2. The prevalence of schizophrenia is about the same in every culture–1 percent.
3. Non-twin siblings show a rate of 10 to 15 percent frequency for schizophrenia; that is, if one sibling is schizophrenic, the other has a 10 to 15 percent chance of being schizophrenic. If identical twins are raised in separate households, and one develops schizophrenia, there is a 40 to 60 percent chance that the other will develop the disease as well.

4. If a child who has no genetic family history of schizophrenia is raised by a schizophrenic mother, his or her chance of becoming schizophrenic is no greater than for the general population.
5. The closer the individual is genetically to a schizophrenic family member, the more likely, on a statistical basis, he or she is to contract the illness. (Goldman, 1988, p. 306)

As can be deduced from this information, there is some sound evidence that schizophrenia is partly an inherited illness.

What is accurate for schizophrenic disorder is even more true for bipolar disorder (formerly called manic-depressive illness), which has a significant genetic base. It is common to see a parent, one or two children, and perhaps grandchildren who have bipolar disorder. But despite the fact that it is quite possible for one to inherit the illness, many escape this fate because not everyone is born with the genetic predisposition. "There remains the possibility that an x-linked gene is a factor in the development of bipolar I disorder in *some* patients and families" (Kaplan, Sadock, and Grebb, 1994, p. 522). In addition, with proper treatment, the illness can be controlled. For example, one of my patients who has a mood disorder has been successfully stabilized on lithium; however, both his father and sister committed suicide.

Studies on the incidence of bipolar disorder in identical twins have strengthened the theory that there is a strong genetic link. When such a trait or illness exists in one twin, there is a 79 percent chance that it will be found in the identical twin. This is called concordance, and appears to occur in high percentages, regardless of whether or not the twins grow up together. In the case of fraternal twins, the concordance rate is about 19 percent (Kaplan, Saddock, and Grebb, 1994).

There are some other psychiatric diseases that also suggest strong genetic origins. Regarding alcoholism, studies indicate that monozygotic twins (identical) show a 26 percent concordance (Goodwin, pp. 427-435). That is, if one twin has the illness, there is a 26 percent chance that the other will also have the illness at some point in time. In the case of dizygotic twins (not identical), the rate is 12 percent.

Similar hereditary factors have been noted statistically in other research studies on alcoholics. It has been shown that if one parent is an alcoholic, there is a 25 percent chance of the offspring having the same illness. If both parents are alcoholics, the rate is as high as 50 percent. Again, the genetic factor seems very strong. One would think that children growing up in an alcoholic home would be totally turned against drinking. However, the genetic influence appears to be very powerful and seems to overcome the adverse conditioning of their childhood.

Research in the anxiety disorders shows less specific genetic tendencies. Clinically, one sees nervousness and worry as familial traits, but statistics do not bear out a hereditary basis for these observations.

Studies in panic disorder specifically indicate that in identical twins there is a 31 percent concordance for the illness. In fraternal twins, however, it falls to 0 percent.

Increasing attention is being paid to these hereditary factors. However, the genetic evidence does not preclude the importance of environmental factors. Stress may often precipitate the development of such disorders.

Though the diseases mentioned may persist because of genetic transmission, treatment with medications appropriate to each disease, along with psychotherapy, can alleviate the symptoms and in many instances allow the individual to lead a productive life. The use of medication will be discussed at greater length in other chapters.

In addition to twin studies and other research into hereditary factors, new work is now being done in genetics. There have been successful attempts to locate genes on chromosomes that are responsible for psychiatric disorders in diseases including Alzheimer's disease, bipolar disorder, Huntington's chorea, diabetes, and Down's syndrome. In the laboratory it has been possible to split genes and recombine them to eliminate the undesirable trait. This is done by injecting a normal gene into bone marrow of the affected animal in an attempt to correct the disease. Such a procedure has actually been done in the case of the Shiverer mouse. This animal lacks the normal covering on nerve fibers (myelin), and has a constant tremor (or shiver, hence the name) that is caused by a genetic abnormality. By replacing such genes, the illness has been cured, and the affected animal eventually develops normal nerve fibers and stops shivering.

Researchers are hoping someday to be able to place normal genes into an embryo or the central nervous system of a person who has a known genetic disorder. By doing this, the normal genes will eventually replace the defective genes, thus reversing the pathology.

These are some of the recent genetic findings in the field of mental illness. These studies will continue, and much more will be discovered. The field is currently in its infancy.

CONCLUSION

The new research on heredity does not deny the importance of a stable home and good parenting. However, it should be emphasized that neither genetic endowment nor parenting are responsible alone for child or adult behavior. Rather, it is the mix of genetics, child-rearing, education, and religious and societal influences that is responsible for the behavior of an individual in his or her society.

The clergy, as well as other counselors, should continually be aware that no single event causes a mental illness, particularly a psychosis or organic mental illness. To blame parents for their children's faults, behaviors, or mental illnesses rarely helps the affected individual. The role of parenting should not be overemphasized, nor should genetic studies be neglected. At the same time, the excesses of our culture (i.e., the proliferation of violence and questionable moral conduct in entertainment, materialism, egocentrism, to name a few) should also not be ignored.

Overemphasizing or blaming any one of these factors for the problems of mental illness is of no help in solving the myriad of difficulties that occur with this unfortunate population. In counseling distressed families, a clergyperson should be careful not to place undue blame on the family for adverse behavior on the part of one of its members.

The cause of mental and emotional illness may never be fully known, but research and time will bring us a better understanding of the complexity of these distressing disorders.

Chapter 3

Biochemistry, Mental Illness, and Medication

The human body contains many miracles. It is so complex that it is doubtful anyone will ever be able to discover all the complex secrets within it. In spite of all the discoveries made thus far, scientists have only scratched the surface of understanding the body. Although it may appear that much has been learned, new ideas and facts about the body are revealed every day. What I learned in medical school about physiology and biochemistry is now being taught in college. The basic curriculum in medical school today includes far more advanced material than it did even ten years ago.

For centuries, man has tried to fathom the mysteries of the mind. Gradually, the enigma has unfolded. The various pathways have been defined, the connections to nuclei traced, and the pathology of diseases described. Neurology and the neurosciences have advanced very far in recent years. The growth in knowledge of the mind's functioning has evolved exponentially. Each year there are new discoveries that add to our knowledge of brain functioning and pathology.

But this is just the beginning of the puzzle. Considering the enormous complexity of the brain, it is not surprising that things can go wrong and that diseases ensue. At the same time, it is amazing that the brain functions so well for so long, often without problems. When watching an Olympic diver or a ballet dancer perform, one cannot help but be amazed by the smoothness of bodily movements. This requires an enormous firing of nerve impulses. In doing so, some nerve cells excite muscles while others inhibit movement. This smooth interplay of muscle movement is only one of the functions of the brain, but it is perhaps one of the easiest to understand. When the brain cells, responsible for the inhibition of muscle movement, are damaged by a disease process, the result is the patient's poor quality of movement. This can best be seen in patients with an illness such as Parkinson's disease, in which there are usually hand and foot tremors and a short, shuffling gait.

Recently, much research has been done on the individual cell. The anatomy, biochemistry, and electrical activity of the cell have been studied extensively. Significant findings on a variety of illnesses have been reported by scientists. Although many physiological mechanisms have been uncovered, such as the role of insulin in diabetes and immunology in infections, there is still a great deal that remains a mystery, for example, the nature of cancer and acquired immunodeficiency syndrome (AIDS).

Although much has been learned about the physiology of the individual neuron, much less is known about the nature of the mind. Although the intact brain is necessary for the mind to function, knowledge of the physical nature of the brain does not necessarily help in understanding the mind. Likewise, information discovered about the mind, through psychological research, does not assist much in the thorough understanding of the brain. Even consciousness is poorly understood. It appears to be uniquely human, and yet consciousness cannot be located in the brain. The famous neurosurgeon, Wilder Penfield, attempted to locate consciousness in a specific part of brain anatomy. But the mind, spirit, and soul of humans are not that easily defined. They are perhaps best understood in metaphorical or metaphysical terms.

WHAT IS A DISEASE?

The modern concept of disease was defined by the German pathologist Rudolph Virchow. He stated that in order to call a physical phenomenon a disease, there must be demonstrable pathology within a cell. Such pathology should be visible by means of gross examination and microscopic examination of body tissue. He asserted that medical scientists cannot call anything a disease unless it can be observed in the pathological changes in cells. In addition, to label something a disease, researchers would have to be able to reproduce the disease experimentally in animals or in humans. For example, if a bacterial infection produces lung pathology, the same disease should occur if the bacteria is introduced in an animal or in another human being. The result would be similar pathology in the lung, both in gross pathology and by microscopic examination. In general, many psychiatric illnesses would not meet the requirements of this definition. Cellular pathology has not been found in patients with schizophrenia, manic-depressive (bipolar) disorder, major depression, or the anxiety disorders.

The fact that cellular pathology cannot be found has led some to perceive severe illnesses, such as schizophrenia, to not be diseases at all. Dr. Thomas Szasz proposed this concept in his book, *The Myth of Mental Illness*. Dr. Szasz contends that schizophrenia is not a disease but rather a behavioral aberration with which society does not cope well. He contends that psychiatrists have a vested interest in hospitalizing patients, and that they make judgments about a patient's behavior, often legally committing patients to hospitals against their will. He further asserts that if individuals are offensive to society (e.g., if they commit a murder), the person should be placed in jail, not a hospital, even if that individual is psychotic. This is certainly a minority view in the field of psychiatry. Most psychiatrists do not see mental illness as a myth. I dare say that this applies equally well to schizophrenic patients and their families. If you had the experience of knowing a schizophrenic person who is a congregant, friend, or family member, you would have great difficulty understanding the individual's behavior as a societal aberration. Recent research has revealed that although there is little visible pathology demonstrable in brain cells with our present laboratory facilities, there are remarkable biochemical changes in patients with schizophrenia and the other major mental illnesses.

Brain Physiology

Much research in the last 30 years has been devoted to brain physiology and the transmission of nerve impulses in the brain. The presumption is that when there is interference in such transmission of impulses from one nerve cell to another, various diseases occur. This implies a new definition of disease as a biochemical disorder rather than cellular pathology.

To understand this phenomenon, it is necessary to review basic brain anatomy and function. This discussion will be far from complete. It is a simplistic view of what happens in the brain. As research proceeds, new biochemical theories will no doubt unfold. The one certain fact to remain is that much of brain pathology will be in the biochemical area rather than on a strictly cellular level.

Each nerve cell (neuron) contains a cell body with a nerve fiber (axon) that transmits impulses *away* from the cell. Another nerve fiber (dendrite) sends impulses *toward* the cell. The dendrites have many spine-like appendages. Through a series of connections, various nerves relate to many other nerves and extend to end organs such as muscles, the heart, the lungs, and the intestinal tract.

The neurons in the brain and spinal cord communicate with each other by meeting at a minute space called a synapse. Here, a chemical exchange occurs, permitting a message or impulse to be carried from one neuron to another. The synapse, then, is a space between the end of one neuron and the beginning of another. The chemicals that are located in the synapses conduct the nerve impulse from one neuron to another. These chemicals are called neurotransmitters. Enzymes also exist in the brain to both synthesize and break down neurotransmitters. Furthermore, substances such as magnesium, calcium, sodium, and vitamins play an important role in the metabolism of neurotransmitters.

There are three main neurotransmitters that are recognized: norepinephrine, dopamine, and serotonin. These naturally occurring chemicals are altered in various diseases. For example, in schizophrenia, there appears to be an elevation of dopamine during acute manifestations of the disease. Medications given for the treatment of the disease lower the level of dopamine in the synapses. As this occurs, the symptoms of schizophrenia tend to lessen or disappear. In depressive disorders, norepinephrine and serotonin are depleted in the synapse, and this corresponds to the symptoms of depression. Antidepressants are used in depression to raise the level of these neurotransmitters in the brain. In contrast, in the manic phase of manic-depressive disorder (bipolar disorder), these neurotransmitters are increased in the synapses. This appears to allow faster transmission of impulses at first, followed by symptoms of mania. In the treatment of manic disorders, medications are used to lower the levels of serotonin and norepinephrine in the brain. As this happens, the symptoms tend to resolve (Goldman, 1988, p. 307).

Thus, the pathology in these serious mental illnesses appears to be in the biochemical area rather than in the structure of the cell itself. As research on the biochemical and metabolic interactions in the nervous system continues, new medications are created to treat the severe mental illnesses that families and mental health workers encounter daily. The stated goal of researchers is to eliminate the disruptive and/or debilitating manifestations of these diseases.

THE USE OF MEDICATION IN PSYCHIATRY

The prolific use of medications in treating psychiatric diseases has existed for only about 35 years. Prior to the 1950s, individuals employed both over-the-counter and prescription drugs for the alleviation of mental or emotional illnesses. Alcohol, nicotine, and caffeine were well-known to affect mood and behavior, and these are still used and abused by many people in the attempt to self-medicate. Morphine, ether, and barbiturate sedatives were also tried by individuals legally or illegally. None of these substances, however, brought about any sustained remissions in patients with schizophrenia, major depression, or bipolar disorder (manic-depressive disorder).

During the 1950s and thereafter, psychotropic or psychoactive drugs were prescribed by physicians to influence the mood, thought, and behavior of the mentally ill. These medications and their mode of action will be specifically described when the various diseases are discussed in later chapters. Generally speaking, there are several types of drugs used in psychiatry.

1. *Antianxiety drugs* are given for short-term improvement of patients with anxiety disorders, including panic and phobic disorders. At times, antianxiety drugs are prescribed regularly for the prevention of these disorders. Such medications are also useful in treating some organic illnesses, including delirium tremors (DTs), which often follow alcohol withdrawal. Included in this group are drugs such as Valium, Librium, Xanax, and Luvox, which is specifically for treatment of obsessive-compulsive disorder.

2. *Antidepressant drugs* are used in moderate to severe depression. When the depression is acute, a remission rate of 60 to 70

percent is common. Medications are generally more successful in treating endogenous depression (which lacks a clear psychological cause) than in treating exogenous depression (in which a distinct external event causes the depression).

Before the antidepressant drugs became available, the only method of treatment for acute depression was electroconvulsive therapy (ECT). In resistant cases and in extremely acute suicidal patients, when several antidepressants have failed, ECT is still administered successfully, usually in a hospital setting. There are various antidepressants that evoke different chemical reactions in the central nervous system. The mechanism of action of these drugs will be discussed later. Elavil, Sinequan, Nardil, Parnate, Desyrel, and Prozac are among the more well-known antidepressants.

3. *Antipsychotic, or neuroleptic, drugs* have been developed to control the various symptoms of severe mental illness. These medications help to alter or eliminate such debilitating symptoms as hallucinations (hearing voices, seeing visions), delusions (false beliefs), or extremely abnormal behavior, such as violent and homicidal tendencies. They are also used to control the heightened and exaggerated behavior of manic patients. Although symptoms are reduced or eliminated, the psychoses are not actually cured by these medications. Recurrences are common. At times, the symptoms do not improve significantly, and a chronic form of psychosis may result in spite of the adequate use of medication. This group of drugs includes: Thorazine, Haldol, Navane, Mellaril, Prolixin, Clozaril, Risperidone, and the latest—the newly released Zyprexa.

4. *Antimanic drugs* are used to treat the acute manic attacks of bipolar disorder and often to prevent recurrence of both the manic and depressed phases of bipolar disorder. Lithium and Tegretol are the most well-known in this group.

SELECTING THE PROPER MEDICATION

When symptoms are mild, most psychiatrists do not prescribe medication. In such instances, psychotherapy alone is sufficient. Once the diagnosis has been determined, based on the patient's history and symptoms, a proper treatment plan can be formulated. If the symptoms are debilitating enough, medication may be necessary. When such a clinical situation exists, the target symptoms of an illness are matched up with the appropriate medication. For example, if a patient is clinically depressed and agitated, the drug of choice would be an antidepressant, which also has sedative side effects that will, in turn, treat the agitation. However, if a patient is moderately depressed and still able to function at work, the preferred drug would be an antidepressant without sedative effects so that the patient will maintain alertness during the working period.

Similarly, the medications needed for the treatment of acutely psychotic patients with delusions (false ideas not found in the patient's culture) or hallucinations (sensory misperceptions where no external stimulus exists) may differ from those used when the patient leaves the hospital. At such time, the symptoms may be considerably lessened or absent. Doses of prescribed drugs must be revised in accordance with the severity of the target symptoms.

It is well-known that patients with similar symptoms vary considerably in their reaction to the same drug. Doses and side effects may differ greatly even within the same group of drugs. It is sometimes necessary to prescribe several medications before the appropriate one is found for a given patient. An occasional patient will not respond positively to any drug. It has been shown by researchers that an antidepressant can be given to patients in a fixed dose, and the patients' blood levels will vary considerably. There are some individuals who can be given huge doses and have a blood level of zero. In such instances, the patient either has not absorbed the drug from his intestines into the blood, or the drug has been broken down in the intestinal tract and rendered ineffective.

The prescribing of medication has its scientific base, but it still remains an art. The careful matching of the most effective drug in a given situation for a specific disease with a particular patient is a challenge for any psychiatrist. Fortunately, the rate of success in alleviating the symptoms of severe mental illness is often high.

Chapter 4

Mood Disorders:
Depression and Manic States

Sometimes people can change quickly. One of your best and most respected congregants may suddenly appear to have too much energy and be acting in a grandiose fashion. You know it; his family knows it; you can tell by his extreme behavior. It really is not like him at all. No one has ever seen him act this way before. Perhaps one of the most helpful women in your congregation, who volunteers for everything and is always there to help others, is gradually slipping into a despondent state. She appears unable to help herself.

What do you do? How do you assess these situations? What help is available? Is this a problem that demands your counseling, or that of a professional psychotherapist or psychiatrist?

In order to know how to approach congregants who have mood disorders, it is very important that the clergy be informed about the essentials of these all-too-common problems. A few general comments about various mood disorders should be mentioned first.

How does the clergyman distinguish between a normal "down" feeling and clinical depression? In dealing with a busy group of congregants, there are signs of lowered ambitions, discouragement, faltering goals and aspirations, which correspond to changes in mood. How does one judge whether these are serious or just temporary changes in mood? In contrast, how does one distinguish between a congregant who has an energetic mood and someone who is manic? In the early stages of mania, this may be very difficult.

First, let us discuss the down side. Generally speaking, if a depressed mood lasts for three to four weeks, it should be taken more seriously; a psychotherapist should be consulted. If the period of depression is abrupt and intense, the affected person should be examined by a professional psychotherapist without delay. Some depressions, when not of a profound nature, can disappear suddenly or after a short period of time. This type may need only brief counseling or interested support from friends, family, and clergy.

When talking with an individual or his family about the onset of depression, the issue of suicide should always be considered. You can ask the questions, "What are your thoughts at the worst time of the day?" or, "Have you ever thought of harming yourself at these times?" If there is any suggestion that suicidal thoughts are present, a psychotherapist should be consulted.

Consider the individual who becomes "high" without the use of drugs or alcohol. At the outset, the person becomes hypomanic; that is, he shows an increased energy level, requires little sleep, and is able to accomplish far more than he normally would. When the pace of the "high" individual becomes frenetic, it can be recognized by anyone as being abnormal. The person will most likely insist that he is fine and that friends and family do not understand him. At such a time, he feels that he can do almost anything, and he becomes irritated at those who stand in his way. Sometimes if the mood progresses, the individual becomes clearly psychotic, and professional assistance is required.

In the following, I will discuss the clinical manifestations of depression and mania and the medical treatment of these disorders. Also included will be some suggestions for the clergy for effectively dealing with congregants affected with mood disorders.

PREVALENCE OF DEPRESSION

It is estimated that in the United States about 9 million persons suffer from depression at any given time. Some experts believe that the number is as high as 15 million. A certain number of these individuals are depressed due to an organic disease, such as hypothyroidism or cancer. (See Chapter 9, "Organic Mental Diseases.")

THE NATURE OF DEPRESSION

What is depression, and how does it manifest itself? Clinical depression is a profound alteration in mood with sadness, despair, feelings of hopelessness, and disturbances in sleep and appetite. It has mental, psychological, and physical effects.

If symptoms are mild, the affected individual usually notices a lowering of mood, some lack of energy, and fatigue with mild sleep problems. Should the depression become more severe, these symptoms progress. The lowered feelings reach a point where the person is unable to respond to his usual interests. Appetite and sexual desire are severely reduced. A weight loss of 20 to 40 pounds is not unusual. Insomnia becomes an increasing problem, with early morning awakening occurring most often. When this happens, the person is not able to return to sleep; worry, anxiety, and restlessness ensue. Loss of concentration and memory are noted by patients. Feelings of worthlessness and guilt and the inability to make decisions are common. I remember a dynamic chief executive of a large company who was so depressed that he was unable to make simple decisions, such as the choice of which clothing to wear or what to eat.

In addition, depressed persons have a feeling of total despair and hopelessness. Suicidal thoughts may occur and attempts at suicide are possible; the clergyperson may be the first to know of the congregant's distress. Since it is very difficult to predict whether someone will attempt suicide, it is best not to deal with this event alone. An experienced psychotherapist should be consulted.

The frequency of suicide in the general population peaks at several different age groups: the first peak occurs in late adolescence and young adult life, between ages 15 to 25; a second peak in the suicide rate is seen in middle age, between 45 to 55; the third peak occurs in the elderly. Recently, studies have shown that persons 65 and over are increasingly prone to suicide, far more than was previously acknowledged. Suicide can also occur in children, although it is uncommon.

When depression reaches the level of symptomatology described here, hospitalization is often necessary to protect the patient from suicide attempts. Since it takes several weeks for most antidepressants to become effective, the patient should be in a controlled environment during the beginning of treatment. If the potential for suicide does not appear imminent, the patient may be treated at home. When depression is acute and treatment is started early, antidepressant medications are effective in treating the symptoms in 60 to 70 percent of cases.

WHAT CAUSES DEPRESSION?

What could possibly cause a person to become so depressed as to slow down physically and mentally to such a degree? Long ago, psychiatrists recognized that some depressions were caused by external events and others seemed to be caused by no obvious factor. These two types were called exogenous and endogenous depressions.

Exogenous depressions are usually precipitated by loss such as the death of a loved one, loss of a job, or loss of power or position. Freud postulated that when such loss occurred, the person was unconsciously very angry about the loss. However, she was unable to express the anger, except to turn it inward; a depressed mood then occurred.

If one is very conscientious, diligent, and somewhat perfectionistic, that person is more likely to get depressed by external forces. Such losses usually cause injury to one's self-esteem, a so-called narcissistic injury.

Endogenous depressions clinically seem the same as the exogenous types; the symptoms are identical. However, the etiology of the endogenous depression is obscure. No significant event of an emotional or physical nature has caused depression. Patients often say, "It came out of the blue." In the endogenous depression, there may be a family history of mood disorder in parents, siblings, grandparents, uncles, aunts, or the extended family; the depression is believed to be more biochemically based. That is, whatever process causes it, the result is a chemical imbalance in the brain that results in depression.

As explained in Chapter 3, "Biochemistry, Mental Illness, and Medication," there is a depletion of the neurotransmitters in the synapses of the brain so that messages that travel from one nerve cell to another cannot be carried with the same speed as normal. Then, a general slowing of reactions throughout the brain and body occurs.

Again, it should be emphasized that even a cursory knowledge of the nature of depression on the part of the clergy is important in understanding the behavior of the depressed individual. All too frequently I have heard the suggestion, usually by a family member, that the depressed person is lazy and unwilling to help herself. When a patient is in the depths of depression, it is virtually impossible for her to function. To call this condition laziness would be similar to asking a man with a fractured leg to run. The clergy can be very helpful in making this clear to the family.

AN ENVIRONMENTALLY INDUCED DEPRESSION: BILL

One day, a new patient, Bill, appeared in my office. He was a 50-year-old married man who had a sudden onset of depression with markedly lowered feelings, hopelessness about the future, and a general slowing down of physical activities (psychomotor retardation).

Bill had always been a hard worker, attended church regularly, and was a "good family man." Now he was unable to work and had lost interest in his previous activities, such as golf and reading. Sleep was often interrupted, and upon awakening frequently at 3 a.m., he was unable to resume sleeping. The idea of suicide came to Bill's mind, especially at these early morning hours, when his mind could not escape the terrible emotional state that plagued him.

This patient was referred by his internist, who could find no physical illness to account for his depression. He had no prior history of depression, nor was there any previous depression in his family. When a patient is this impaired, it is of little value to discuss in detail the origin of the depression; that is, to try to uncover what might have been the precipitating factors. In this condition, most patients can not concentrate enough to deal with such issues; it is better to wait until the patient has improved.

I decided to begin treatment with a combination of psychotherapy and an antidepressant medication. I saw Bill twice a week in my office since I was satisfied that he was not a serious suicide risk. He was also given a sedative to help him sleep.

After about two weeks the patient was sleeping better, and he felt that he was at least not deteriorating mentally. Bill's mood gradually improved, as did his appetite. In the fourth week of treatment, Bill began to think about the possibility of returning to work, which he was able to do on a part-time basis. Two months later he announced that he was 80 percent improved, and after six months, he was totally functional. At this point, the dose of medication was gradually reduced and then eliminated.

This patient revealed, in a humorously sardonic way, that when he was in the depths of despair, he would have given me all of his possessions—his home, both cars, his bank accounts, everything he held dear, excluding his wife—if I could have promised him full recovery from his pain. However, he added that now that he was feeling well, he resented paying my modest fee.

As he began to feel better, I inquired into possible emotional and environmental causes for the onset of his depression. This particular patient had problems asserting himself; he usually got along with others because of his mild and ingratiating manner. Before the onset of his illness, Bill encountered a new supervisor who was arrogant and intimidating. Bill's natural manner and defenses could not deal with the situation, and he became withdrawn and depressed.

A psychodynamic view of this man's problem would be the following: the patient's angry impulses were clearly in conflict with his superego (conscience). His ego could not find an appropriate manner to deal with the situation. He felt *hurt* instead of angry. He unconsciously turned the anger inward against himself, rather than expressing it outwardly.

In the process of psychotherapy with this man, I tried to help him understand that he had to modify his passive nature and deal more appropriately with confrontation. We discussed the ways in which he handled anger. As a religious man, he felt it was sinful to get angry at anyone, regardless of the circumstances. I pointed out to him, in a variety of ways, that anger had its usefulness and that it could be used appropriately either as an expression of true feelings or in ways that were inappropriate and, perhaps, even immoral.

We talked about expressing feelings in an effective manner so that the other person could understand his feelings and what his position was on any given issue. He began to understand that emotions are important, and that the expression of feelings is valid. He realized that in some instances it required more responsibility to express feelings openly than to conceal them. This appealed to his conscientious side.

After about one year of psychotherapy, long after he had stopped using medication, Bill was able to adequately deal with and have a working relationship with his boss, which did not adversely affect him in an emotionally distressing way.

In such instances, the psychotherapist helps the patient to gain insight into his typical patterns of behavior. By acting as an emotional catalyst, the psychotherapist attempts to alter the patient's former inadequate methods of dealing with his environment.

In addition, when the patient gains awareness to the etiology of his illness and determines the emotional dynamics that cause depression, he or she can often prevent recurrence of the symptoms. This is the most valuable aspect of psychotherapy with exogenous depressions.

A BIOLOGICALLY INDUCED DEPRESSION: BOB

There are episodes of depression that occur without a clear-cut psychological reason. A person may be feeling well and may be able to carry out his daily pursuits in the usual way, and suddenly, within days, may become acutely depressed. This does not mean that there are no psychological factors involved, but rather that they play a minimal role. The following case is an example of this type of depression.

Some years ago, I received a phone call from a 45-year-old executive named Bob. He told me that he was having great difficulty getting up in the morning to go to work. He said he had been depressed for about two months and was feeling worse every day. When he came to my office, I could see the distress on his face. He moved slowly and spoke with considerable hesitation. He complained of black moods; a lack of concentration, especially at work; insomnia; and some memory problems. Although he was not suicidal, he did express feelings of hopelessness about his illness.

This man was very upset because the depression had happened twice before. The first episode was mild and occurred while he was in college. He could not recall any events at that time that might have triggered the depression.

Bob's second bout with this illness came when he was 35 years old. At that time, he had been rising rapidly in his professional career, had gotten married, and had one child. He felt that his life was in order, and he could not identify any reason for his mood change. Although there had recently been some added stress at his job, it was not of the nature that would ordinarily bother him.

Inquiry into Bob's family history revealed problems with mood disorders in his father and uncle. Both had recurring bouts of depression and had been hospitalized and given electroconvulsive therapy.

I began treating Bob with antidepressants. It took a long time for his symptoms to respond to the medication. Finally, he began to show some change. Meanwhile, I had to assure him that most depressions do diminish and disappear in time. It took some months before he was fully restored to health.

Because of the recurring nature of his illness, the lack of clear precipitating events leading to his depressions, and the strong history of depression in his family, it was my assessment that he was suffering from a more biologically determined illness. Accordingly, I recommended to him that he be placed on a maintenance dose of lithium, which is known to prevent future attacks of recurrent depression. It has been ten years now since I first met Bob, and he has remained on lithium; Bob has been free of any symptoms during this entire time.

In such cases, many patients on lithium feel increasingly confident in their ability to avoid depression because they feel so well. It happens frequently that the patient, inspired by such feelings, will stop taking lithium. Sooner or later, the depression returns. After one or two such relapses, most patients are convinced that they require lithium maintenance to remain well.

People often view depression in simplistic ways. All of us have the human tendency to label and pigeonhole things or events. It enables us to codify and simplify the vast amount of information that comes to us daily. By eliminating much of the data that is available to us and accepting only that information that confirms our initial prejudices, we ease our mental work and arrive at simple answers. This organizing proclivity is capable of making us radicals, arch conservatives, racists, and bigots. It can also lead to the gross oversimplification of our view of emotional illness. As examples, frequently heard statements about depression are the following: "People who get depressed are just feeling sorry for themselves," "They don't want to get better," "They just have to think positively." Obviously, those who make these statements have never experienced the feelings of utter helplessness that accompany the depressed person's condition.

In order to understand mood disorders, some description of the different manifestations of these illnesses is helpful. The following classification of mood disorders is condensed from the *Diagnostic and Statistical Manual* (DSM-IV), published by the American Psychiatric Association.

Mood Disorders

Depressive Disorders

1. *Major depression*–This is a severe depression, occurring in a single episode or in a recurrent form, usually years apart. It may be precipitated by environmental stressors or be of the endogenous type.
2. *Dysthymia (or depressive neurosis)*–This is a mild to moderate depression that, by definition, must be at least two years in duration. It is believed to be due to external causes, presumably from neurotic conflicts.
3. *Depressive disorders not otherwise specified*–These are atypical depressions that do not fit the previous definitions. An example from this group is the recently recognized depression that is affected by the seasons of the year. It is called seasonal affective disorder (SAD). Typically, its onset is in the fall, and it tends to disappear in early spring. Patients with this form of affective disorder respond well to artificial light, which can prevent the depression.

Bipolar Disorders

Bipolar I Disorders

These may include single or recurrent episodes, manic or depressed phases, or a "mixed" condition in which both manic and depressive stages occur. In the manic mood, the patient has an unusual amount of energy. He or she sleeps only a few hours per night, goes on wild spending sprees, and has delusions of grandeur, such as being a great inventor, musician, a savior, etc. If untreated, the patient can become overtly psychotic. At such times, it may be hard to distinguish the illness from schizophrenia. In the depressed phase, the patient has the usual symptoms described earlier. The manic or depressed phases may last for weeks or months. The intervals between episodes may last for months to years.

Bipolar disorders are now believed to be largely hereditary in nature although environmental influences can help to precipitate an attack.

Bipolar II Disorders

In this condition, there are recurrent depressive moods along with intermittent hypomanic episodes. The latter are mild manic attacks rather than full-blown manic states.

Cyclothymic Disorders

Both high and low moods occur in this condition. They are clinically less severe and often are not treated because the symptoms are mild. Nevertheless, it can be a very debilitating illness. When depressed, the patient does not function well and is very distressed. When in a hypomanic state, the patient is hard to live with, as he may be overactive, argumentative, arrogant, and quite unlike his usual self.

Bipolar Disorder Not Otherwise Specified

This category is used when the illness is atypical and does not fit any other classification.

Mood Disorder Due to a General Medical Condition

This includes a substance-induced mood disorder. Some other medical conditions that can cause a mood disorder include the following: hypothyroidism, hypoglycemia, tumors of the adrenal glands, and brain tumors.

MEDICAL TREATMENT: ELECTROCONVULSIVE AND ANTIDEPRESSANT THERAPY

Only 35 years ago, there was no way of treating the depressed or manic patient, except with the use of electroconvulsive therapy (ECT) or by simply sitting out the disease. Although the very thought of electroconvulsive treatment brings terror to the minds of most people, it has been a very effective therapy. In very resistant cases, it is still used when drugs fail to help the patient.

How is ECT administered and is it dangerous? Before using this procedure, the patient is usually examined by an internist to determine whether there is any physical disease that contraindicates the use of this treatment. Serious heart disease, brain tumors, and a history of stroke are considered reasons to avoid its use.

In most cases, the patient is now treated in a hospital setting. An anesthesiologist is present to begin the procedure. He or she inserts an intravenous tube and administers a sedative anesthesia similar to that used in gynecology for a uterine scraping (D&C). It is mild anesthesia, but sufficient for the patient to be completely unaware of the treatment. The patient is also given a muscle relaxant to prevent a typical grand mal epileptic seizure. By so doing, when the electrical stimulus is given, the seizure that is experienced is reduced to fluttering of the eyes, facial twitching, and slight contractions of the hands and feet. After the seizure, the anesthesiologist assists the patient with breathing and awakens him or her. Usually within 10 or 15 minutes, the patient is able to walk unassisted to ward activities. There is a temporary loss of memory for the time just before and after the treatment. The treatment is repeated three times per week for 4 to 12 treatments until the patient improves. ECT is now a very safe and effective treatment. Death occurring from its use is extremely rare and is much less frequent than from general surgery.

There are times when ECT is still the only way to prevent a patient from committing suicide or to help him through a serious depression. Most psychiatric hospitals continue to use ECT in a judicious manner. Despite the positive results and relative safety of ECT, there are groups still very much opposed to the use of this type of therapy.

ANTIDEPRESSANT MEDICATIONS

In discussing the use of medication for mood disorders, it should be kept in mind that the psychiatrist must be very supportive and, indeed, therapeutic in dealing with patients who require medication. There are some physicians who prescribe antidepressants without any concurrent psychotherapy. It is my conviction that this is improper; depressed patients need much support due to their emotional pain and the possible risk of suicide.

There are presently several categories of medications that are used in the treatment of depression. They include the tricyclic antidepressants (TCAs), the monoamine oxidase inhibitors (MAOIs), and a miscellaneous group. The largest category is the TCAs, which refers to the group's three-ring chemical configuration. They are chemically related to the antipsychotic drug Thorazine.

The Tricyclic Antidepressants (TCAs)

In 1957, a compound called imipramine was first found to have antidepressant properties. It has since been used as a standard antidepressant against which others are measured. Imipramine was first marketed as Tofranil.

The following is a list of the commonly used TCAs:

- Elavil, Endep (amitriptyline)
- Asendin (amoxapine)
- Norpramin, Pertrofrane (desipramine)
- Sinequan, Adapin (doxepin)
- Tofranil (imipramine)
- Aventyl, Pamelor (nortriptyline)
- Vivactil (protriptyline)

As previously indicated, the level of neurotransmitters in the brain appears to be lowered in depression and elevated in manic states. Antidepressant drugs tend to raise the level, resulting in clinical improvement. Usually, 10 to 14 days are required for this to begin, and maximum improvement occurs in six to eight weeks.

The exact nature of the biochemical changes that occur is unknown. The neurotransmitters–norepinephrine, serotonin, and dopamine–relay messages from one nerve cell to another. They are continually being produced, used, and eliminated. Tricyclic antidepressants are believed to prevent the normal uptake or elimination of the neurotransmitters, thus causing a rise in their level in the synapse and restoring them to normal amounts. Another theory involves the effect of antidepressants on increasing receptor sensitivity, which presumably normalizes the transmission of cell impulses. It is also theorized that the endocrine system contributes to the development of depression. Symptoms, such as weight changes, insomnia, and altered sexual interest, all of which are controlled by the endocrine system, are clearly observed in patients with depressive disorders.

When neurotransmitters at the base of the brain in the hypothalamic-pituitary area are lowered, clinical changes associated with depression can result.

Common Side Effects of Tricyclic Antidepressants

Most side effects in this group of medication are due to anticholinergic (blocking the brain's acetylcholine) effects. These result in symptoms such as dry mouth, constipation, and swelling of the extremities. Effects on the heart include rapid heart rate and palpitations. Difficulty with close vision (such as reading) and an adverse effect on certain types of glaucoma are possible. Rarely, a paralysis of the small intestine and inability to begin urination has been observed. As with all drugs, allergies can occur.

In rare instances, tremors, problems in muscle coordination, and weakness can occur. The potential for these side effects increases with age. Hence, the elderly can only tolerate lower doses, but the therapeutic effect in this age group is similar to younger patients.

Side effects can be reduced by lowering the dose or switching to another class of antidepressants. Generally, if one class of antidepressants does not help a patient with depression, another class of antidepressants may be effective.

Monoamine Oxidase Inhibitors (MAOIs)

This group includes the following:

- Parnate (tranylcypromine)
- Nardil (phenelzine)

The enzyme monamine oxidase is present in the brain to slow down the activity of neurotransmitters. Specifically, it deactivates the neurotransmitters norepinephrine, dopamine, and 5-hydroxytryptophan. MAOIs all inhibit monoamine oxidase, thus allowing an increase in neurotransmitters.

This type of antidepressant, as with so many findings in the field of medicine, was discovered quite by accident. In the 1950s, there was still a high incidence of tuberculosis. A drug called iproniazid was commonly used for this illness. The physicians and staff, in institutions where it was administered to patients, noticed a distinct elevation in mood in patients who previously had been depressed. Iproniazid was later used in controlled studies with large groups of depressed patients. The results were positive in a high percentage of cases.

The MAOI antidepressants were marketed extensively until some patients were found to have developed unusually high blood pressure spikes, resulting in severe headaches, and on rare occasion, in strokes and death. Researchers discovered that a substance called tyramine, found in certain foods, in combination with the MAOI, produced this dangerous effect. Aged cheese and meats, wine, beer, etc., contain high amounts of tyramine. When these foods are eaten while a patient is taking an MAOI, adverse reactions may occur. If the patient excludes these foods from his diet, the drugs can be taken for depression and used safely and effectively.

In practice, TCAs are generally prescribed first. If they prove to be ineffective, patients are given one of the MAOI antidepressants.

Common Side Effects of Monoamine Oxidase Inhibitors

The most common side effect of these drugs is postural hypotension (feeling lightheaded or dizzy when changing positions from lying down or sitting to standing). Other side effects such as dry mouth, constipation, delayed urination or ejaculation and impotence can occur, but these are uncommon. Liver damage, although quite rare, has been reported in some patients.

As mentioned, severe headaches, high blood pressure, and possible intracranial bleeding (stroke) can result from the simultaneous use of these drugs and foods containing tyramine.

Newer Antidepressants

In recent years, several antidepressants have been synthesized in the hope of finding drugs that either have fewer side effects or are more useful in treating patients unresponsive to TCA or MAOI drugs. Two such newer medications are Ludiomil and Desyrel. They are chemically different from those already mentioned, are equally therapeutic, and have similar side effects. Desyrel is believed to have less influence on heart rate although it causes more drowsiness.

Prozac is a new antidepressant that is now available for depressed patients. It has been hailed as the new miracle drug. As with all such "miracles," it takes several years to see whether it is as helpful as it is purported to be. It has the advantage of not causing marked weight gain in patients, it does not produce drowsiness, and usually only one dose is required daily, as a rule. Generally, there are few side effects. Recently, there have been several law suits by patients claiming that the drug made them violent and more suicidal. Research over the last three to four years has discounted these findings. To date, about 8 million patients have been given the drug, and only a few bad reactions have been claimed. I have had some positive results using this new drug for depression.

Among the most recent selective serotonin reuptake inhibitors available for depression are Zoloft (sertraline) and Paxil (paroxetine). These drugs are of similar effectiveness to Prozac.

USING ANTIDEPRESSANTS
IN OTHER PSYCHIATRIC CONDITIONS

As mentioned, many discoveries in medicine are accidental. So it was with the revelation that certain antidepressants were of some assistance in patients with chronic pain. Small doses of these drugs, taken with traditional pain medications, are more helpful in relieving pain than when only pain medication is used. An antidepressant such as Elavil has had a positive effect on pain, whether the source of the pain is muscular, nerve related, or chronic in nature.

Panic attacks, particularly those associated with agoraphobia (fear of leaving the familiar setting of home), have been reduced or eliminated by small doses of tricyclic drugs.

One young man I treated had severe agoraphobia. He was only able to shop in a nearby store and drive his car in his neighborhood. If he went beyond a certain area, he developed severe panic. On a small dose of Tofranil he was able to drive almost anywhere that he wished.

Manic Behavior

As noted above, an individual can show manic symptoms alone, or he or she can go through cycles of manic and depressed behavior. The manic phase was already described, but here is an example of what is commonly observed by psychiatrists in patients that have manic attacks.

One day, I received a call from the wife of a 45-year-old executive. She said that he had been behaving strangely for some time. At first, he became more energetic than usual. Both she and her husband saw this as a positive change, since prior to this time Joe had been procrastinating and allowing his work to go uncompleted.

But Joe began to have still more energy; he worked 16 hours a day, required little sleep, and did not have time to eat. She became very concerned when he bought two new cars without telling her, and then charged over $10,000 to their credit account in a short period of time without discussing it with her. This was not like him at all. She asked him to talk with their pastor or a local physician, but he refused. He simply said that he felt fine: "Why should I ask anyone for help when I am feeling so good?" One day, he came home and announced that he had invented a new computer. This seemed unreal to his wife since he had only an elementary knowledge of computers.

By the time Joe was brought in for treatment, he had lost 25 pounds, looked tired, but was still going strong. He very reluctantly agreed to go into a hospital for treatment. This happened only after his wife threatened to leave him if he did not go. (In dealing with mania, a firm approach is one thing that seems quite useful.) Sometimes, behavior becomes so extreme that the family cannot cope with the patient and the police have to be called in to deal with the situation.

After several required laboratory tests were done, Joe was placed on a major tranquilizer to calm him. He then was given increasing doses of lithium for his mania. After about one week, he was much calmer and realistic about his abilities. His judgment improved significantly; he appeared normal in his behavior as well as in his expressed ideas. I informed him that he had to continue to take the lithium or he would quite likely experience another attack of mania. He found this hard to believe. Most manic patients, upon recovery from the first attack, do not immediately become believers in the medical treatment of this disease. Usually, it takes two or three similar episodes to convince a patient that this is an illness, and that treatment for it exists. Better still, there is a way of preventing the illness by the regular use of lithium or another drug (Tegretol or Depakote). Successful treatment requires the psychiatrist to persistently educate family members and patients to convince manic patients to continue to use these medications.

A LOOK BACKWARD

I remember all too well the time before antidepressants and lithium were available for the treatment of mood disorders. Trying to conduct psychotherapy with a deeply depressed person was a difficult and frustrating experience. Session after session, the affected person would repeat his or her symptoms: the hopeless feelings, insomnia, poor appetite, loss of weight, and other reactions typical to depression. All that a psychiatrist could do, aside from ECT treatments, was give the patient support and perhaps a sleeping pill, and wait out the depression. This could take as long as nine months to a year.

The clinical use of the antidepressant drugs for depression has made a remarkable difference in treatment. It could be compared, in some ways, to the use of antibiotics in the treatment of infection.

Instead of waiting for the natural history of the disease to unfold, the duration of the illness is sharply curtailed; this allows the patient to return to normal activities much sooner, thus avoiding regression to less functional states. In a similar way, lithium has been effective in preventing mania and depression. All this has made the psychiatrist's task in treating the mood disorders much easier. However, there are still some psychotherapists who believe that psychoanalysis is the only long-term answer to depression; they refuse to use medication. As a qualified psychoanalyst, I believe that in so doing, these psychotherapists may cause unnecessary suffering for the depressed person in the service of their own favorite theory. They prolong the depression and even risk the possibility of suicide. Tracing the origin of a deep depression using psychoanalysis is best done after the depression has been alleviated. The same could be said for manic behavior. In the case of endogenous illnesses, however, this is often difficult to do.

HOW CAN THE CLERGY HELP?

It is at the onset of acute mania or depression and after the hospital stay that the clergy can be very helpful. At the beginning of the manic episode, the family needs much support in recognizing the illness and dealing with the affected person.

In contrast to other mental illnesses, when a family member experiences a manic high, it is surprising what a friend or outsider can do to influence him or her. The clergy can be very instrumental at such times in suggesting that help is needed. Likewise, after the initial attack has subsided, the clergy can be very supportive in reminding or even convincing the patient that the use of continued medication is necessary. Such reinforcement by others can make the psychiatrist's work more effective and, of course, make the patient's life happier and more productive. If you, in your role as a cleric, assist a family in this way, the patient's family and your congregant will both be very grateful to you.

In a paper I wrote a few years ago, I discussed how in an inner city environment, persons afflicted with mania often allow the illness to progress much further before being brought in for treatment. Abnormal behavior is tolerated more in the large cities, and families are often more dysfunctional. As a result, patients are less restricted in their behavior and are not readily recognized as behaving abnormally. This results in symptoms similar to those mentioned, followed by much more severe manifestations, such as delusions (ideas of grandeur) and less often, hallucinations. I have seen inner-city clergy be of great assistance in bringing their disturbed congregants to the hospital for help. Additionally, there are other ways that the clergy can help congregants who are subject to mood disorders.

The more you know about the extremes to which moods can go, the better you will be in recognizing when you can play a significant role. I would like to emphasize the fact that all moods are not the result of external stresses. It is very tempting for one to see all mood changes as originating in events occurring in the person's life. There may be other causes of severe mood changes, such as drugs or organic illnesses.

As noted, the length of time and the degree of mood change that occurs is very important in determining what the clergy can do. It is at the early stages and after recovery that the clergy can be of greatest assistance. Reassuring the patient, counseling the family, and encouraging the proper use of medication as prescribed can all be of enormous help to the patient.

If there is any hint of suicidal thoughts in a congregant, a mental health professional should be consulted immediately. It would be unwise to try to counsel such individuals or to attempt to only use spiritual assistance to help them "pray their way out of it." I have seen several religious individuals wait months and even years while praying for their depression to end. These people could have received help sooner and consequently could have led productive lives for those months. This is not to deny the efficacy of prayer, but rather to include all the additional services one can provide in addition to offering spiritual help.

When in a depressed mood, patients often experience much associated guilt. Such feelings are not generally based on any real wrongdoing on the part of the patient. Rather, guilt is known to be part of clinical depression. If any slight wrong had been done, it may be grossly exaggerated during a depression. When the patient has recovered from his deep, depressed mood, he will regard the perceived wrong in the proper light. As mentioned in another chapter, delusional guilt may also occur. For example, a person may feel that he has caused another to become very ill just by having had some bad thoughts about him.

In these situations, the clergy can be very helpful in assisting a congregant to become aware of the exaggerated nature of expressed guilt. At the very least, the clergy cannot add to the problem by treating the guilt as a reality-based issue. Also, when talking to a depressed congregant, the clergy should be aware that a quiet, confident voice can be very reassuring to someone in the depths of despair; simply listening to a depressed congregant can provide great comfort and security.

In dealing with patients who are experiencing a mental illness, I have always been aware that a psychiatrist or any other psychotherapist cannot do his or her work in isolation. Friends, relatives, clergy, employers, and others can all be either very helpful or injurious to the distressed individual. The thought has occurred to me on many occasions, "I will take all the help that I can get." This certainly includes the clergy.

In the field of family therapy, such joint assistance has been emphasized considerably. That is, patients do not live in isolation, but rather in a system. Everything and everyone in that system affects everything and everyone else. When the persons in a given system act conjointly to help a distressed individual, it is much more effective than when attempts are made by one person alone. Having said all this, I must also ask the clergy to consider when they are helping too much. I refer you to the writings recently published on codependence. There are times when we, in the helping professions, do more harm than good by overdoing the helping role. It appears that even counseling can be overdone. I will discuss this in more detail in Chapter 8, "Alcoholism and Drug Abuse."

Family members often criticize a depressed person as being lazy. The physical and mental slowing so characteristic of depression can create this appearance. But far from being lazy, the impaired person is truly unable to do normal expected tasks. However, as improvement occurs, the individual can do more if firmly encouraged. The clergy should advise family members of this situation. Depressed congregants do not need lectures on being lazy or uncooperative; they need sympathy and firm support.

It has been my impression that the role of the clergy in the support and help of the mentally ill has been grossly underrated and ignored. I further feel that religion and the work of the clergy hold society together in a way that is not fully appreciated in this modern scientific era. There is a great need for psychotherapists to appreciate the role of the clergy. Likewise, the clergy can work very cooperatively with professional psychotherapists in better helping ailing and distressed congregants.

Chapter 5

Schizophrenic Disorders

When I first saw the young woman, she was quiet, withdrawn and isolated. Although originally a good student, she gradually lost interest in school. She no longer had friends and was not active in her former pursuits. Her affect (feeling tone) was dull, but her mind was sharp. She could remember things well; she could calculate and answer questions relevantly. However, there was much missing. There was a hollowness about her, a failure to respond emotionally, and a distance in her gaze that her family had not seen before.

As time went on, she spoke very little and became somewhat incoherent. Gradually, she deteriorated and required hospitalization. While this appeared to be a quiet and deceivingly benign onset, it represented a serious illness with a bad prognosis. It was one form of schizophrenia–the disorganized type–that will be discussed in more detail later.

Another patient whom I saw some years ago was a 15-year-old high school student, who began to have delusions that she was destined to become a famous musician. She could not play any instrument and planned no music lessons, but that did not deter her from her goal. She also had very unrealistic ideas about what she could do to help others understand world problems and provide for world peace. She was not setting realistic goals and spoke as though she had already reached these ambitions. Such grandiose ideas are sometimes associated with manic behavior and sometimes with schizophrenia. As time went on, it became apparent that she had a schizophrenic disorder.

Another patient, age 18, had a sudden onset of paranoid ideas, although he previously appeared to be quite normal. He thought that the police were after him and that signals were coming to him from outer space. He was convinced that his radio was instructing him to hide. Such delusions can be very frightening and can lead a person to drastic action. Persons so afflicted with paranoia can be schizophrenic, but it is also possible that they might be reacting to street drugs, such as speed, cocaine, marijuana, LSD, and other substances. There are many physical illnesses, such as hyperthyroidism and arteriosclerosis that can also cause paranoia.

These examples describe a few ways in which schizophrenia can make its appearance to a family. Often, in their confusion and concern, families will come to clergymen or clergywomen for help. In such situations most clergy would immediately recognize the severity of the presenting symptoms, and refer their congregant to a local physician or directly to a psychiatric facility. Failure to do so would delay treatment, compromising the outcome and creating needless havoc for the patient and his family.

WHAT IS SCHIZOPHRENIA?

If you ask the average person this question, the answer would be: "It's a split personality." That is not correct. The term "split personality" refers to the diagnosis multiple personality disorder. It is a neurotic disorder and has nothing to do with the psychosis schizophrenia.

Schizophrenia has long been an unsolved puzzle to the medical community. This disease shows remarkable changes in thinking, feeling, and behavior. There occurs a splitting, not in personality, but in the functions of the mind; however, the personality can often deteriorate in the process. For example, abilities such as memory, calculating, and other cognitive functioning may remain intact, while the individual has delusions and/or hallucinations (hearing or seeing things that others cannot perceive). Emotions often seem very inappropriate to the expressed thoughts. Frequently, considerable withdrawal from people and a flattening of affect occurs.

Behavior can range from regression to childhood, with symptoms of wetting and soiling, to paranoid ideation. A patient may respond to a hallucination, such as a voice instructing him to kill himself or someone else. In many forms of this disease there is a thought disorder, in which logical thought breaks down and the patient has ideas that are loosely associated. That is, she fails to make sensible connections between thoughts or even words. Other symptoms can occur such as mutism, in which the patient does not communicate at all. Various mannerisms and stereotypical behavior (movements or posturing) are seen.

Although schizophrenia usually begins in adolescence or young adult life, the American Psychiatric Association states in its *Diagnostic and Statistical Manual* (DSM-IV) that it can begin as late as age 45.

There are two main forms of schizophrenia. One type begins gradually and insidiously, continuing on a downhill course. This type tends to have a very poor prognosis. The first example mentioned in this chapter is an illustration of such a case. This condition is regarded as being more constitutional or genetic in nature, rather than being caused by environmental stressors.

The other form of schizophrenia has a more acute onset, is of shorter duration, and resolves much faster, often without any residual symptoms. The case of paranoia mentioned above is representative of this type. Environmental stressors are believed to play a much larger role in this form of schizophrenia.

Currently there are five types of schizophrenia, as noted in the DSM-IV classification. They are as follows:

1. *Catatonic type*–In this condition, the patient shows marked stupor, a lack of spontaneous movement, a decrease or lack of verbal communication, negativism, and stereotypical behavior. Patients may also demonstrate a condition called "waxy flexibility," in which the patient's arm can be moved to any position and will remain there for hours. A variation of this type is the excited patient, who shows increased motor activity and purposeless movements. This form may be very dangerous to others. Some patients may suddenly and without warning go from the quiet, stuporous type to the excited type. It is at this stage that the patient may become markedly destructive.

2. *Paranoid type*–This is perhaps the most familiar presentation of this disease in which the patient is very suspicious and has delusions (false beliefs). He may receive messages from the radio and television (ideas of reference), or he may feel that

the FBI is after him or someone is plotting to kill him. He may feel that others are putting thoughts in his mind or that he is able to put thoughts in the minds of others. In addition, hallucinations may occur. The feeling tone is usually appropriate to what the patient is thinking or saying.

3. *Disorganized type*—Here, there is a gradual onset, as in the first case discussed. There is a marked disturbance in behavior and a severe thought disorder in which the patient is very difficult to understand. In addition, the patient may regress to childhood and become very silly, laugh inappropriately, or show a very flat affect (emotional tone).

4. *Chronic undifferentiated type*—This type is a general category that does not fit the other more specific descriptions. There are marked delusions, frequent auditory hallucinations, occasional visual hallucinations, and a very marked deterioration of behavior.

5. *Residual type*—In this type, the acute symptoms such as hallucinations, delusions, and incoherence are diminished and not as prominent. However, many abnormal behaviors remain, such as a flat affect, inability to work productively, social withdrawal, lack of initiative, and some forms of thought disorder.

A BRIEF HISTORY

Schizophrenia has been known for many centuries. Ancient writers referred to it often and described its various bizarre manifestations. It was viewed, variously, as a disease of the brain, devil possession, or an unusual spiritual state. Accordingly, it was dealt with by physicians and clergy, depending on the period of civilization and the culture in which it occurred.

The history of psychiatry is replete with unusual stories of how schizophrenia was handled. It was not until the eighteenth century that the French physician, Philippe Pinel, took the mentally ill out of the dungeons and chains, placed them in suitable quarters, and treated them psychologically. This was the beginning of more humane care of the mentally ill.

An interesting book by Dr. Benjamin Rush, a physician who practiced during the days of the American Revolution, describes the early treatment of the mentally ill in hospitals. The care of the mentally ill was surprisingly advanced, even though it included such old practices as cold water baths and bloodletting to treat insanity. But it was not until recently that there was any method of successfully caring for and rehabilitating the mentally ill, of which patients with schizophrenia comprise the largest group.

It should be noted that in the 1940s, 50 percent of all hospital beds in the United States, including medical, surgical, pediatric, and other categories, were occupied by mentally ill persons. Most of these were schizophrenic patients. Today, because of antipsychotic drugs, that number has been reduced to 25 percent (Goldman, 1988, p. 305).

WHAT CAUSES SCHIZOPHRENIA?

The exact cause of this disease is not known. There are hereditary factors as well as environmental causes. As indicated previously, the various manifestations of the disease depend on which of these play the more important role. Research indicates that 1 percent of the population is subject to schizophrenia.

Although many stressors have been implicated as causes for precipitating the disease, none have proven to be specific. At one time, inadequate mothering was blamed. Poverty, inner-city crowding, poor education, vitamin deficiencies, and many other causative factors have been investigated. Although there is no denying that the above factors can play a role in mental health, they do not specifically cause schizophrenia.

There is good evidence that hereditary factors play an important part in the occurrence of the disease. As discussed in Chapter 2, "Parents, Society, and Heredity," if one parent has schizophrenia, the incidence among the children is about 10 to 15 percent. If both parents are schizophrenic, the number increases to 30 to 50 percent. This occurs regardless of whether the children are raised with their parents or with foster parents. There is also a much higher incidence of schizophrenia in identical twins if one of the twins develops the disease (Goldman, 1988, p. 307).

In the families of schizophrenics there is also a greater tendency for family members to show signs of alcoholism and antisocial behavior; however, the incidence is not remarkably above the rate for the general population. It is not known whether this is related to genetic factors or has some other cause.

ANTIPSYCHOTIC DRUGS (NEUROLEPTICS)

It was not until the 1950s that medications began to be used in the treatment of major psychiatric illnesses such as schizophrenia, manic-depressive disorder (bipolar disorder), and other psychotic behaviors, regardless of cause. The medications used for these disorders are variously called antipsychotics, neuroleptics, or major tranquilizers. For discussion purposes the term antipsychotic will be used to indicate these drugs.

In 1954, Dr. Nathan Kline reported from Rockland State Hospital in Orangeburg, New York, that a drug called reserpine, had antipsychotic properties. Reserpine was isolated from the Indian snakeroot plant. It had been used in India for high blood pressure and for sedation. Dr. Kline treated a large number of schizophrenics with reserpine, and the treatment proved to be successful. At about the same time, a drug called Thorazine was synthesized. It also had antipsychotic properties, but it was more effective.

Mechanism of Action

Thorazine and the other antipsychotic drugs that were subsequently developed work basically by antagonizing the neurotransmitter dopamine. In schizophrenia, there is an excess of dopamine in the brain, which presumably causes the symptomatology. Thorazine blocks the transmission of dopamine to receptors in the synapses, thus eliminating the acute symptoms of the disease. The exact mechanism is probably far more complicated, and it is being extensively explored by researchers.

Classification of Antipsychotic Medication

There are a number of antipsychotics on the market consisting of different chemical classes. They are all effective, and the psychiatrist's choice of drug is determined by such factors as the stage of the disease (acute or chronic), the side effects of the drug, and the physician's familiarity with a given drug. The following is a list of some commonly used antipsychotic drugs. Brand names are followed by generic names in parentheses.

- Thorazine (chlorpromazine)
- Mellaril (thioridazine)
- Serentil (mesoridazine)
- Trilafon (perphenazine)
- Stelazine (trifluoperazine)
- Taractan (chlorprothixene)
- Navane (thiothixene)
- Haldol (haloperidol)
- Loxitane (loxapine)
- Moban (molindone)
- Risperdal (risperidone)
- Zyprexa (olanzapine)

Treatment with Antipsychotics

All these medications have been used extensively for the treatment of schizophrenia, particularly in acute-care settings. High doses are prescribed until symptoms are under control. Lower doses are used for maintenance therapy in outpatient settings.

Schizophrenic patients are often treated in community mental health clinics, where a wide variety of treatment modalities are used. Group and individual therapy, activity therapy, and vocational and housing assistance are provided by such clinics, along with the required medications.

Unfortunately, there has been insufficient funding by communities and states for such clinics. The result has been massive discharge of patients from state and county hospitals, with insufficient community programs to assist patients. This inequity is one of the serious social and medical problems our nation must face. It is estimated that the majority of homeless persons in this country are suffering from some form of mental illness, and services for them are sorely needed.

Psychiatrists in private practice also treat schizophrenic patients with or without the concomitant use of community mental health clinics.

Although medications have allowed many patients to leave hospitals and return to the community, some schizophrenic patients do not function well. Although many return to previous levels of functioning, others show marked regression and deterioration. Unfortunately, the treatment of schizophrenia, although improved, has not reached a level of cure.

The more acute symptoms of schizophrenia, such as delusions and hallucinations, usually resolve quickly with the use of antipsychotic drugs. In some cases, in spite of adequate medication, the patient continues to experience these symptoms in a chronic, although less intense form.

Patients with the more chronic form of schizophrenia show considerable withdrawal and flattening of affect. Antipsychotic drugs do little to help these symptoms, and the latter may remain persistently as negative symptoms. However, a new drug named Clozaril (clozapine) has been recently approved for treating schizophrenia. It promises to significantly affect these negative symptoms. However, it has been known to have one serious side effect, namely, agranulocytosis, a condition in which the white blood count drops to dangerous levels. This makes its use limited to certain patients who have not benefited from any other medication. These individuals need to be closely monitored for changes in their blood counts on a weekly basis. If the white blood count drops below the normal level, the drug is discontinued, and serious complications are avoided.

Side Effects

Antipsychotic drugs have a number of significant side effects. The most common are disturbances in motor function in the so-called extrapyramidal area. This part of the brain is responsible for the smooth and delicate coordination of muscle control. Without such inhibitory effects on muscle activity certain symptoms can occur, such as the following:

Akinesia—A reduction in voluntary movements, this side effect results in a lack of facial expression or a loss of normal swinging of the arms while walking.

Akathisia—In this state of motor restlessness, the patient finds it difficult to sit still and often paces or wrings his hands. Insomnia may also occur.

Dystonic reactions—The sudden involuntary spasms of certain muscle groups, usually in the neck, jaws, larynx, or the muscles that control eye movements. Because of the suddenness of onset and lack of voluntary control, these side effects although uncommon, can be very frightening.

Pseudoparkinsonism—This syndrome resembles Parkinson's disease, which is common in the elderly. Muscles become rigid and weak. When resting, there is a rhythmic tremor of the hands. When walking, the patient may take short steps while leaning forward. Sometimes the patient finds it difficult to stop. There may be a jerking motion of the arms and legs. Normal arm swinging, while walking, does not occur.

Tardive dyskinesia (TD)—As a result of chronic use of antipsychotic drugs, some patients develop tardive dyskinesia. It usually happens after a patient has been on drugs for several months or years, and it occurs in about 10 to 20 percent of patients who require long-term care. This syndrome may involve abnormal movements of the lips, facial tics, grimaces, or abnormal chewing movements with protrusion of the tongue. These symptoms do not necessarily disappear if the drug is stopped. The syndrome can be quite disabling and disfiguring. Chronic long-term use of antipsychotics and high doses of the drug appear to be positively related to the occurrence of the disorder. Unfortunately, there is no known cure; researchers are attempting to find medications that will reverse these abnormal movements.

Controlling Side Effects

Aside from tardive dyskinesia, the other abnormal side effects mentioned above can be controlled in several ways:

1. The dosage of the drug can be reduced.
2. The physician can substitute another antipsychotic drug.
3. Tolerance can develop in some patients over time.
4. The use of anticholinergic drugs such as Cogentin and Artane, or antihistamines, such as Benadryl, can combat the side effects of antipsychotic drugs. They are variously effective and seldom eliminate the side effects completely.

How Antipsychotic Drugs Are Used in Treating Schizophrenia

A 25-year-old man named Joe was brought in by his parents because of unusual behavior. For some months he had been withdrawn, had not gone out to see friends, and had missed work. When asked by his family why he was doing this, Joe replied that he was tired. His former delight in reading had disappeared, and he had become overly engrossed in television. Finally, he was unable to work at all. When observed, he appeared to turn his head, as though listening to what others could not hear. He began to speak of the government sending out the FBI to check on him as he thought he was suspected of having committed crimes, which he denied doing. Joe was afraid to eat because he thought that the food was poisoned. Consideration had to be given to the possibility that this young man was abusing drugs. When this was ruled out with a drug screen and by consulting with his family, a diagnosis of schizophrenia, paranoid type, was made.

The symptoms described are very typical of a first episode of schizophrenia. Before the antipsychotic drugs were used, such a patient would have had a 50 percent chance of relatively full recovery after six months of hospitalization—usually in a state hospital. The same results can now be obtained in a higher percentage of cases within several weeks of treatment with neuroleptic medications.

Let us return to our patient. Joe was placed in a psychiatric unit of a general hospital. I prescribed the drug Navane 10 mg four times a day. He developed stiffness of his arms and legs and restlessness. I gave him Cogentin to relieve these side effects. In three weeks, he was no longer paranoid, nor was he hearing voices; his former interests returned.

Upon leaving the hospital, Joe was able to function well with a reduced medication plan without the use of the Cogentin. For the next two months, he was on Navane 5 mg three times a day. On this dose he was sent back to work. Gradually, the medication was reduced further, and after six months he was off all medication.

Meanwhile, Joe was seen on a weekly basis for psychotherapy. Some of his acknowledged stress at home and at work were discussed. The patient was given emotional support and encouragement when needed. I made no attempt to analyze the patient to determine why he had had a psychotic episode. In the movies and in television programs, any psychiatrist worth his salt would not have been satisfied with such a recovery until he had unearthed the underlying problem. One reason for not doing so is time constraints. But, even if the patient and the psychiatrist had unlimited time and motivation, it would still be very difficult to determine the reasons for a psychosis occurring. This has been attempted in long-term care in certain hospitals in this country and elsewhere, with the results sparse and not very satisfactory. For an account of such treatment by a psychoanalyst, I refer you to the book by Joanne Greenberg, *I Never Promised You a Rose Garden.*

There are no studies of which I am aware that indicate that such long-range use of psychotherapy, without the use of antipsychotic drugs, is in any way better than the use of these drugs and supportive psychotherapy in treating schizophrenia. Certainly, cost factors are greatly increased in the long hospitalizations. Also, prolonged hospital stays can have a deleterious effect on patients when they are deprived of work and interaction with friends and family.

The patient described here did well, and in the ten years since his illness began, he has not had a relapse. In cases in which such relapse does occur, the same basic treatment would be carried out, but the medication would probably be used for a longer time, perhaps one to two years with weekly, biweekly, or monthly psychotherapy sessions.

If patients do not recover fully from the acute manifestations of their illness, it may be necessary to give medications over a long period of time. In such instances, it is usually beneficial for a patient to attend group and individual sessions at a community mental health center, if one is available in the patient's area. Some patients also find assistance and solace in a national organization called Recovery. This self-help group is run by patients according to principles established by Dr. Abraham Low in his book *Mental Health Through Will Training.*

Research efforts continue in the direction of finding improved antipsychotic drugs that have fewer side effects and greater efficacy in treating the varied syndromes of schizophrenia.

Meanwhile, the families of the mentally ill, including schizophrenic patients, have organized a group called the National Alliance for the Mentally Ill (NAMI). It is dedicated to raising funds for research. Their goal is to eradicate mental illness through research into hereditary, environmental, biological, and other factors that may be responsible for these diseases. This highly motivated group, now consisting of over 150,000 members, has been very active in working with the psychiatric community to reach their mutual goal of eliminating mental illness.

THE ROLE OF THE CLERGY

In every religious group, whether it be at a temple, church, or other religious institution, there will be congregants suffering from some form of schizophrenia. The clergy can be very helpful to the families of schizophrenics, as well as to the patients themselves. In the town in which I live and work, one of the churches has organized and supported a social group for these mentally impaired individuals. They meet weekly, have dinner together, and talk about their problems. Such groups are very supportive to those involved and make the difficult lives of these patients more bearable.

But even on an individual basis, the attention of a clergyperson to such persons can be enormously effective. The role should be primarily one of support. When a crisis develops, a member of the clergy may be the first one to whom the family goes for support and guidance.

If the clergyperson has even a rudimentary knowledge of schizophrenia, he or she will be able to feel more at ease with such afflicted persons. Working with both patient and family can be a very gratifying experience to any member of the clergy, but it requires reaching out to help these unfortunate individuals. Let me suggest the following:

1. *Educate yourself about the illness.* This can best be done through the national organization that was created by the families of the mentally ill. This group is called The National Alliance for the Mentally Ill. Through its newsletters and recommended reading, it disseminates information on the latest findings on the research and treatment of schizophrenia.

2. *In talking with schizophrenic patients, use simple communication.* Long dissertations on any subject will be poorly comprehended. Avoid the use of highly symbolic language or metaphors. When giving instructions, keep the ideas simple and direct. Write down suggestions for your congregant, so that he or she can refer to them in your absence. Failure to transfer your ideas in writing may result in the listener forgetting your thoughts.

3. *Call the schizophrenic congregant on the phone periodically.* These folks are very lonely and isolated. A phone call may mean far more than it would to another of your congregants. While you are talking to him, encourage the person to take his medication on a regular basis.

4. It has been observed that when emotions in a family are dramatic and highly expressed, the schizophrenic patient does poorly. When the family is able to reduce the expressed emotion to a normal amount, the patient does far better. *The clergy can help by counseling the family to try to keep the emotional level subdued.*

To those who have not tried to work with the mentally ill before, I would strongly recommend such an experience. Again, this should be in a supportive role along with the proper psychiatric care.

Chapter 6

Other Psychotic Disorders

There are several psychoses that are classified in the DSM-IV with "Schizophrenia and Other Psychotic Disorders." Since they are relatively common, they require further discussion.

The first of these is delusional disorder. This mental illness may have a sudden onset or begin insidiously. It consists of persistent paranoid delusions such as being followed, poisoned, or deceived or any other paranoid idea. The person may respond to these ideas and direct her life in accordance with these delusions or do very little else other than harbor such notions in her mind. By definition, the condition has to be at least one month in duration. Patients with this condition seldom have hallucinations, which differentiates this illness from schizophrenia. Bizarre behavior, thought disorder, and inappropriate affect, commonly seen in schizophrenia, are also absent.

The delusions in this disorder may involve grandiosity, pathological jealousy, feelings of persecution, erotomania (i.e., a person of a higher socioeconomic plane is in love with the subject), or the belief that they have a dreaded disease.

Patients with this disorder may have difficulty trusting others, have low self-esteem, and be hypersensitive. Feelings of resentment and a tendency to blame others are common in paranoid individuals. Little is known about the cause of this illness.

Formerly this disease was referred to as paranoid disorder or paranoia. The latter diagnosis was reserved for the condition in which a delusional idea was the predominant feature of the disease, while the rest of the personality and intellectual functioning remained intact. Paranoia is now included under the heading of delusional disorder.

SCHIZOPHRENIFORM DISORDER

In the past, this disorder was not distinguished from schizophrenic disorder. The symptoms of each are identical, but in the case of schizophrenia, the course is long and usually chronic. By definition, schizophreniform disorder is less than six months in duration. There may be only one episode in a lifetime, or there may be repeated episodes with interludes of normal behavior. Some of these patients may subsequently develop schizophrenia or another illness such as bipolar disorder. Those with very short-lasting illnesses have a better prognosis, but if the course lasts almost six months, the possibility of schizophrenia resulting in the future increases.

To illustrate, a patient named John came to see me about a marital problem. He was 55 years of age and told me that when he was 25 he had a sudden onset of a psychosis that lasted for about one month. At the time, he was delusional and was hallucinating. He was hospitalized and diagnosed as schizophrenic because that was the diagnostic trend at that time. He never had a subsequent psychotic illness. By the current definition, he was not schizophrenic; he had, however, lived his intervening life thinking of himself as schizophrenic and fearing that he would have another breakdown. I have seen other patients who reported transient psychoses lasting several days. These episodes were clearly schizophreniform in nature and had no organic cause. There may not be any precipitating event that precedes the illness, and the exact cause of the disease is not known.

SCHIZOAFFECTIVE DISORDER

This diagnosis is reserved for those patients who show a combination of schizophrenic symptoms and a mood disorder. That is, in schizophrenic disorder there are no primary symptoms of an affective disturbance, and in bipolar disorder, in which the mood is primarily altered, there is no thought disorder, withdrawal, or blunting of affect as seen in schizophrenic disorder. In schizoaffective disorder, the symptoms appear at the same time.

This diagnosis is generally used when it is very unclear whether either of the two primary diagnoses is prevalent. At the present stage of classification of diseases, this diagnosis is somewhat vague and is not made very often.

BRIEF REACTIVE PSYCHOSIS

The hallmark of this psychosis is that an unusual precipitating event heralds the onset of the symptoms. The event may be loss of a loved one, a severe accident, or a disaster. The psychosis is sudden in onset and usually brief in duration, lasting less than a month. The symptoms are acute, and hallucinations, delusions, disorganized thinking, and confusion may be present. The illness apparently occurs more often in persons with borderline and histrionic personalities.

In contrast to the other major psychoses, this illness is believed to be caused by psychogenic factors rather than biologic or organic causes.

INDUCED PSYCHOTIC DISORDER

In this condition (also called shared paranoid disorder), the person living with a family member or friend shares the same delusional beliefs. The first member is usually more psychotic than the other. The persons are very dependent on each other, and one is more dominant. This disorder may occur between two persons or more. The most extreme example of this was the Jonestown disaster, in which a large number of persons committed suicide because of shared religious beliefs dictated by their leader. The more common presentation of this illness is found within a family, between two people, and most often between sisters (Goldman, 1988, p. 329).

PSYCHOTIC DISORDER
DUE TO A GENERAL MEDICAL CONDITION

With this classification, the medical condition is specified. A further distinction is made as to whether there are delusions or hallucinations present.

TREATMENT OF THE PSYCHOSES

If the symptoms of a psychosis are mild and it is possible to treat the individual at home, the psychiatrist can prescribe antipsychotic medications. These drugs are both sedating as well as helpful in resolving the psychotic symptoms. If the patient is out of control, he may require hospitalization. This can be comforting to the individual because it temporarily removes him from the stressful situation and provides for his needs while subduing disturbing symptoms. In either the office or hospital setting, the psychiatrist usually engages the patient in supportive psychotherapy. Some of the illnesses described in this chapter are brief reactions, and the person will return to normal functioning after a short interval. The delusional disorder and the shared delusional disorder tend to be much more resistant to treatment.

THE ROLE OF THE CLERGY

In these disorders, the main features are psychotic symptoms. These illnesses resemble schizophrenia and the severe mood disorders. The role that the clergy can play is likewise similar to the suggestions made in the chapters on these separate major illnesses: Chapter 5, "Schizophrenic Disorders" and Chapter 4, "Mood Disorders: Depression and Manic States."

Chapter 7

The Neuroses

In the current classification of the neurotic disorders in the DSM-IV, there are three basic groups.

1. anxiety disorders (anxiety, phobic neuroses)
2. somatoform disorders
3. dissociative disorders (hysterical neuroses, dissociative type)

ANXIETY DISORDERS

A young, healthy-looking man walked into my office appearing quite distraught. He seemed fearful and agitated. "How can I continue working in New York, when I can't cross the bridge to get there? I'll lose my job. What will I do with my family? I'm going to be a failure!"

The symptoms began suddenly and without warning. One day, while riding the bus across the George Washington Bridge, Josh looked out of the window and saw the water below. He had done this many times before and never experienced any foreign sensations. This day, however, he felt absolute panic. His heart was pounding; he began to perspire, and he felt like he had to get out of the bus. He tried desperately to stay in his seat and managed to do so until the bus had reached the New York side. He then got out in order to try to calm himself. After about 20 minutes, Josh felt better, but he began to think about how he was going to get home again. This created another wave of panic, but not to the same degree as he had previously experienced.

Thoughts began to creep into his mind: "Am I having a nervous breakdown? What if this gets worse? Will I end up in a mental hospital like that guy at work?" He walked around for a time, and then decided to call home. His wife tried to assure him that he would be all right. He had severe doubts about that. When she offered to pick him up, he welcomed the suggestion.

Oddly enough, on the way back, Josh had very little discomfort while going over the bridge. He wondered how that was possible. It was the same bridge. He was just going in the opposite direction.

Josh's wife talked with him at length, and she felt that he should talk with a doctor about it. He went to see his internist, who examined him, found no physical disorder, and made the diagnosis of anxiety disorder. He prescribed a tranquilizer and told him to try returning to work the following day. Josh, who was not one to be easily thwarted, gave it "the old college try." It was a disaster! Finally, he was sure he was going off the deep end so he called his doctor again, who recommended that he talk with a psychiatrist. This confirmed Josh's worst fears; he really was a "nut"–absolutely crazy and headed for a mental hospital.

When he came into my office, he said that he was a wreck from all the worry and concern. After hearing his story, I assured him that I had never seen anyone go to a mental hospital for the type of symptoms that he was experiencing. He found this hard to believe, but tried to accept my statement as true. I suggested that he get himself under control by allowing the weekend to pass, while taking a sufficient dose of medication to relieve his anxiety.

My plan for treatment was to attempt to understand the basis for the sudden onset of his anxiety, and simultaneously, to get him back to work as soon as possible. The latter proved to be the easier of the two. With a sufficient amount of medication, he was able to make it across the bridge, but not without considerable discomfort. When he arrived at work, he felt somewhat better knowing that the return home would not be as difficult as the morning trip.

As I got to know Josh, I discovered that he was quite successful at his job, but recently he had encountered a new situation that was very different from anything that he had previously confronted. One of his clients was a very aggressive, demanding, and overbearing person. While trying to handle him in his usual agreeable style, Josh noted that this man made him very anxious. Josh did not associate the problem with his client to his panic on the bridge, but the two were related. After some discussion, it became clear that he was suppressing his contempt for his client because he wanted to maintain the work relationship.

In therapy, I tried to help Josh deal with his present crisis in a constructive way without feeling intimidated by his client. I also made him aware of the historical roots of his problem; the lack of aggression was related to his overbearing and dominating father. By confronting his immediate source of anxiety at work and taking a more assertive position with his client, he began to feel more in control of the situation rather than the victim of the interaction. This, in turn, relieved his "bridge" symptoms, and he was gradually able to feel much more comfortable. In such cases, symptoms are apt to return unless the patient is able to recognize the emotional problems, understand the origin of the symptoms, and try to alter his life so as to avoid further problems.

What Are Anxiety Disorders?

Anxiety is a generalized, very unpleasant feeling of apprehension. It is often hard for the patient to describe. It is usually accompanied by physical discomfort such as palpitations, shortness of breath, excessive perspiration, and motor restlessness. Although it occurs in many forms, it is usually sudden in onset and not clearly related to a given cause. As a result, there are mild to moderate difficulties with reality testing and interpersonal relationships. Most psychotherapists, except behaviorists, believe that anxiety is caused by a psychological conflict that is largely unconscious.

Anxiety disorders differ from personality disorders in that the latter represent a life-long pattern of maladaptive behavior that is not as likely to bother the person who has the disorder. Rather, individuals with personality disorders are often quite annoying to those around them. In contrast, persons who suffer from anxiety symptoms are themselves quite troubled by their illness. Most of us have neurotic symptoms at one time or another that may not be severe enough to be classified as a disorder. Probably everyone has had anxiety on some occasion.

It is estimated that about one-third of the general population suffers from an anxiety disorder at some time. Certainly, the number of persons that are impaired by these conditions is high. "The

Age of Anxiety" is a common term used to refer to the current American culture. The anxiety level does not appear to be decreasing.

How Do Anxiety Disorders Develop?

Before the turn of the century, Freud wrote about a new illness that he called the *anxiety neurosis*. He began his work with the study of hysteria, the common syndrome that occurred at that time. Many patients, especially women, had conversion reactions such as paralyzed limbs, psychological blindness, or inability to speak. These infirmities were not based on any physical pathology.

In Paris, Freud worked with another physician named Charcot, who had a clinic for patients suffering from these illnesses. The only known treatment for hysteria at that time was hypnosis. Freud used this form of therapy extensively, but he observed that although patients' symptoms would disappear with hypnosis, they soon reappeared. He postulated that a force was present in the mind to make this happen. Through the process of free association and the analysis of dreams, he was able to detect conflicts within the patient's mind that were not obvious in ordinary conversation. Freud argued that because the patient was unable to tolerate certain wishes, he or she repressed these thoughts and this resulted in symptoms. All this occurred without the patient being aware of the process; it was done unconsciously. In effect, the mind had its own way of dealing with conflicts between the id (basic drives) and the superego (conscience). It all happened through the use of defense mechanisms.

What Is a Defense Mechanism?

It is a process by which unacceptable impulses or wishes are unconsciously managed by the mind in order to prevent anxiety. A good example of this is the defense called repression, which I like to view as unconscious forgetting. In the example of the man with the bridge phobia, the patient first tried to repress his anxious feelings, but without success. He then displaced the fear of his client onto a fear of the bridge.

Note that a bridge is a significant symbol, as it gets a person from one place to another. "Bridging the gap" is a phrase we often use in a variety of contexts, not the least of which is the "gap" between persons. Freud felt that the patient's phobia represented or symbolized an important concept to the patient. In addition to repression, displacement, and symbolization, most persons, who suffer from phobic disorders also use the defense mechanism of avoidance. The following diagram will help to explain Freud's concept of how anxiety disorders develop.

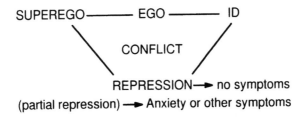

A conflict between superego and id results in the defense mechanism of repression, in which the conflict is suppressed to the unconscious level. Most of the time, when conflicts occur, repression is all that is needed. If repression is only partial, anxiety neurosis or another form of neurosis may result.

In the example of the patient with the phobic disorder, several other defenses were unconsciously playing a role, namely, displacement, symbolization, and avoidance. Instead of anxiety, the defense mechanisms resulted in a phobic disorder. Freud postulated that an illness, such as a phobic disorder, would be much easier for the individual to tolerate than a continual state of anxiety.

There are a number of other defense mechanisms, some of which I will define. All operate in an unconscious manner.

Acting out–Instead of reacting to feelings in one situation, a person inappropriately responds to these feelings in another situation. If a boy is angry at his parents, he may not express this directly but may break a school window or begin to shoplift.

Conversion–Rather than experiencing anxiety, the mind converts a conflict to a physical illness involving the voluntary muscles or the special senses. Symptoms may include pain, paralysis, or loss of a sensory function such as sight or hearing.

Compensation–With this defense, the person tries to compensate for what is unconsciously felt to be his inadequacies. Constant bragging in an attempt to cover up deficiencies is a common example.

Idealization–A person exaggerates or overestimates qualities that she highly regards in another individual.

Identification–Unconsciously, the person adopts the qualities of someone else. If this is done on a conscious level, it is not defined as identification but rather as imitation.

Isolation–With this defense, ideas and feelings are separated from each other, thus allowing thoughts to be present in the mind without the memory of accompanying uncomfortable feelings, which were associated with earlier experiences.

Intellectualization–Information and reasoning are used instead of a person feeling emotions that are appropriate to a given situation. When asked how one feels about a friend's death, the person does not reveal feelings at all but is apt to relate a textbook account of how the death occurred.

Projection–Using this defense, the individual unwittingly blames others for things for which he is partially responsible. If one cannot accept feelings of hate within one's self, he or she may become deluded into thinking that others hate him or her.

Rationalization–A socially acceptable reason is offered for the real one. When arriving late for work, it is "because of the traffic." This is not a conscious excuse but rather an unconscious process.

Reaction formation–A fear of an unwanted impulse is replaced by its opposite. Excessive caring may be a substitute for wanting to reject or hate another person.

Regression–With this defense, one moves to a more primitive form of behavior in an emotional sense, in physical or emotional illness, or even in everyday activities such as play or sleep.

Sublimation–In this defense, unacceptable emotions are rejected and are deflected into socially approved behavior. Rather than overtly expressing anger toward someone, the person may divert his or her energies in an aggressive sport.

Undoing–The impulse to do something and its opposite impulse may occur in rapid succession when a person is using this defense. In compulsive hand-washing, the impulse to have done something bad is symbolically removed by the washing.

In discussing the various anxiety disorders, somatoform disorders, and dissociative disorders, I will illustrate how these defenses are used.

There is no one who escapes at least some form of anxiety in life. Everyone has neurotic conflicts. Anxiety disorders (formerly called neuroses) are but an exaggerated state of the conflicts within us all. When these conflicts, to which we are all heir, become highlighted in our lives and impair our functioning, then they are clearly recognized as neurotic.

Panic Disorder

It came on suddenly and without warning. My patient was sitting high up in the stands of the football stadium. He loved the game, and seldom missed an opportunity to cheer on his team. But, today it was a different story. For no apparent reason, he felt strange physical sensations. He began to shake, had palpitations, had shortness of breath, felt nauseous, and thought he was having a heart attack. There was no way he could stay to watch the game. His friends took him to a nearby hospital emergency room. After careful examination and testing, the doctor told him that he had no physical signs of heart disease or any other pathology. He called it a panic attack.

Such panic attacks are not uncommon and occur much as just described. They can happen with or without agoraphobia. The latter is a fear of leaving a safe place because of the possibility of a panic attack occurring. It is a fear of being in areas where there might not be any escape (caught in traffic, crowds, far away from home). In recent years, agoraphobia has become more prevalent, perhaps because people travel more frequently and farther from home than ever before. Often, the greater the distance from home, the worse are the symptoms of agoraphobia. As the individual begins to travel toward home, the panic gradually subsides.

I have known patients who have been literally housebound for years because of the fear of panic attacks or the associated agoraphobia. One of my patients with these symptoms finally had to leave home because of a physical illness and was forced to go to an emergency room at a local hospital, thus breaking the long-standing isolation from the outside world.

In order to prevent the symptoms of panic disorder and agoraphobia, most people will use the defense of avoidance. They simply will not leave what they regard as safe, i.e., home. Psychotherapists use the term "separation anxiety" when referring to the fear patients have of leaving secure places or persons, where safety and comfort are paramount. Such anxiety usually begins early in life whenever a youngster is separated from home or family. It is common in so-called "school phobia," which is usually caused by a fear of leaving home.

There is also a strong tendency toward using the defense of regression, in which the patient retreats to earlier and more primitive forms of behavior. Thus, seeking the safety and security of home and of persons who are emotionally close becomes very important.

Social Phobia

Suffering from this disorder, the individual is very shy and fearful of social situations. There is an acute sense of embarrassment or a fear of making mistakes, eating in public places, and exposing oneself to ridicule. Again, the defense of avoidance is used extensively. As a result of the illness, there can be a severe limitation to the person's experience. This prevents emotional and psychological growth and creates low self-esteem.

Simple Phobia

The bridge phobia previously described is a good example of this type of phobia. It can involve fear of heights (acrophobia), water (hydrophobia), fire (pyrophobia), closed spaces (claustrophobia), pain (algophobia), fear of dirt and germs (mysophobia), fear of strangers (xenophobia), and many other phobias. The defenses used in phobias were previously illustrated. Certainly, avoidance is the most obvious defense in this illness.

Obsessive-Compulsive Disorder

This is an illness that may contain one or both aspects: an obsession and/or a compulsion. An obsession is a recurrent thought or idea which is difficult to control. Although it may not make sense to the person afflicted with it, there is a preoccupation with the symptoms, which is very distracting. It is sometimes impossible for a person to rid herself of these thoughts. For example, I have treated mothers who had recurrent thoughts about harming their children. These thoughts were completely contrary to any real intention on the part of the mothers who were, without exception, very conscientious women. Also, the recurring thoughts of doing harm never resulted in any injury to the children. It was a true obsession. (Parents who abuse their children seldom have any obsessive thoughts about it.) In treating these patients, I found that they had considerable anger toward someone else—anger that was not recognized or expressed. When this was brought to the patient's awareness and handled appropriately, the obsession disappeared. In most instances, this was accomplished in a relatively short time, perhaps six months.

But there are more severe forms of obsessive-compulsive disorder. Every psychiatrist has treated patients with compulsive hand-washing tendencies. One of my patients had to clean his hands 20 times before going out of the house. After urinating, the hand-washing had to be repeated. If he tried to wash only ten times, he would experience considerable anxiety. Sometimes the obsessive-compulsive behavior takes up most of the patient's day. It also is very frustrating to those who are living with him or her.

Persons with this disorder have a hard time expressing their emotions. They use several defenses in order to avoid coming into contact with their conflicts and attendant emotions. One of these defense mechanisms is intellectualization. For example, if one were to ask such a person how he *feels* about a recent friend's death, the reply will often be a quote from a doctor or a reliance on statistics rather than an expression of feeling.

Another defense common to this disorder is called isolation. Using isolation, the person detaches his or her emotion from the original source of memory that caused a conflict. In this way she does not have to experience the conflict again.

Still another defense frequently seen in this disorder is called undoing. In this defense, the person ritualistically repeats a behavior in order to avoid anxiety. The act is usually highly symbolic. The best example is compulsive hand-washing.

Although trained as a psychoanalyst, I have found that applying the analytic method to these problems is very time-consuming and not always helpful. I like to try behavioral methods first or in conjunction with more analytic methods.

For example, I examined a man named Jack who had an obsession with cleanliness. Although he was unusually concerned with his house being orderly and neat, this was no problem to him as his wife preferred it that way, too. But, what she could not tolerate was his cleaning up after her, and especially his half hour showers and ten-minute hand-washing rituals.

From an inquiry into the patient's background, I learned that Jack was a very successful, hardworking man who had no complaints about his life except for his compulsions. He managed his interpersonal relations at his job satisfactorily although some of his colleagues wondered why he washed his hands so much. The fact that others knew about his symptoms troubled him more than anything else. His personality was rigid and he had difficulty expressing emotion—a typical obsessive-compulsive personality. I elected to try a behavioral technique called desensitization. I asked Jack to decrease his hand-washing. That is, instead of 20 times, I told him to try washing 19 times and to experience the anxiety that followed and try to cope with it. After a short time, he was able to do this. Simultaneously, I asked him to go into his backyard and muddy himself with dirt and water. Although very reluctant to do so, he managed to accomplish this task on occasion.

When first in private practice, I saw a young child who regularly soiled her pants. She was very compulsive, even at the age of five. Much of the soiling behavior stopped by the regular use of finger painting, which I encouraged at home as well as in my office. This technique was similar to the "muddying" idea used with my adult patient.

Gradually, Jack was able to decrease the hand-washing to a more reasonable level. While desensitizing him, I also discussed his need to express his feelings more. However, his rigid personality would not allow any real emotional changes, and he did not have much interest in pursuing long-term psychotherapy.

In treating obsessive-compulsive symptoms, there is no reason why psychodynamic therapy cannot be used along with behavioral techniques or with the simultaneous use of medication, when it is indicated. This is called multi-modal treatment (Lazarus).

Post-Traumatic Stress Disorder

A traumatic stress is an unusual event such as a serious harm to family members, a community disaster, a violent accident, or wartime calamity. Following the event, the person reexperiences the episode in some way. This can happen by recall, dreams, or a sudden feeling that the event is recurring; it can also be set off by incidents that remind the individual of the original trauma.

The syndrome includes the avoidance of anything that is related to the original trauma as well as some failure to remember significant parts of the trauma. There is a "psychic numbing," that is, an inability to experience normal emotions and a general detachment from those who were close. In addition, persons suffering from this disorder may have sleep disturbances, anxiety, and problems with concentration.

This condition was first recognized during World War II. It was referred to as shell shock or war neurosis. At a certain point during the severe stress of active combat, the individual stopped functioning and had to be taken to the back lines for evaluation. He appeared in a daze and was often brought back to reality by medical hypnosis. This was accomplished by the intravenous injection of sodium amytal and the suggestion that the person talk about and express emotionally–abreact–what he had experienced. Although this procedure was temporarily useful, the whole syndrome of post-traumatic stress disorder often followed.

In some instances, even years later, the trauma would be reexperienced. I can recall a young man who, as a child living in Holland during the war, endured the trauma of frequent bomb attacks by the German Luftwaffe. Years later as an adult, he often had nightmares about the bombing. He was known to scream loudly, awaken his family, and usually have no recollection of the experience. If awakened during the nightmare, he would recall that the disturbance was due to his early traumatic experience. Many Vietnam veterans have this disorder. In recent years it has been recognized as a syndrome that can result from any unusual trauma; it is not confined to the horrors associated with war.

A number of methods have been used to treat post-traumatic stress disorder. Individual and group psychotherapy, medication, and hypnosis have all been useful, particularly when combined in a treatment plan. Hypnosis by an experienced person and medical hypnosis are both effective in helping the individual recall and reexperience the original trauma. Psychotherapy is useful in coping with the remembered material. Medication may help the accompanying anxiety.

Generalized Anxiety Disorder

In this condition, the anxiety is the main feature. For a patient to be diagnosed with this disorder, excessive anxiety must be present for at least six months. It can become chronic and last for many years. The amount of anxiety is not appropriate to the events of the person's life. Worry, apprehension, increased physical tension, and overactivity of the autonomic nervous system are present. The latter produces palpitations, difficulty breathing, increased perspiration, abdominal distress, and many other physical symptoms. In addition, there is hypervigilance, insomnia, and problems with concentration.

Sometimes severe anxiety can be confused with physical diseases such as hyperthyroidism, hypoglycemia (low blood sugar), and neurological disorders. It is very important that a physician examine such a person to rule out any disease that may be present.

Let me illustrate. One day I was discussing a sexual problem with a young married couple. It was arduous because the young woman was very inhibited and had difficulty revealing her feelings about the subject. She appeared so nervous and upset that I asked her how she felt physically. She was having palpitations and was light-headed. I took her pulse; it was 120 beats per minute. I interrupted the session and called her internist. He was able to examine her within the hour. She had a sinus tachycardia (abnormally rapid heart beat), which needed treatment. It became clear that physical and emotional problems were going on simultaneously. It was important to first manage the physical problem before continuing with the psychological difficulty. Handling one without the other would have been inappropriate.

SOMATOFORM DISORDERS

Body Dysmorphic Disorder

This disorder is a condition in which there is a great preoccupation with a physical defect in a person who appears normal or who has a slight defect that would ordinarily be ignored.

The woman who appeared in my office one day was extremely attractive by any standard; however, she had an excessive concern with the appearance of her nose. She was convinced that it was asymmetrical. To the casual observer, she had no such defect. However, when she went to great pains to show me what she meant, it became apparent that if one were to measure both sides of her nose with a micrometer, there might be a perceptible but very minimal difference. In her mind, however, it was immense and was responsible for her failure to become a more successful model. Similarly, many individuals have a preoccupation with being "hippie" when their hips are small or fat when they are slender. These are distortions in body image. Some feel that a body part is too big or too small, even though it could not be confirmed by unbiased observers. I love the T-shirt emblazoned with the saying, "No body's perfect, but some of my parts are excellent." In a humorous way, this exemplifies a healthy attitude toward physical imperfections. As a 35-year-old patient said to me, "I had a beautiful body until I turned thirty. After that, it was all maintenance." Her wry comment was reminiscent of the usual complaint about an aging automobile.

Body dysmorphic disorders are not easy to treat. Patients who have this problem hold on to their complaints tenaciously. It serves as a defense against facing reality in their lives. Dealing with these realities may be too difficult to bear. Being obsessed with a physical defect is not unlike obsessive concern with a mental problem. Since there is such a need to maintain the symptoms, the individual is often impatient with treatment, does not face reality, and quits treatment prematurely.

Conversion Disorder

In Freud's era, this illness (also known as hysterical neurosis, conversion type) was as common as phobic disorders are today. It occurred especially in young women. A sudden attack of paralysis, deafness, inability to speak, or other unexplained physical illness left the patient helpless. The symptoms were confined to the voluntary motor system (muscles) or the special senses (hearing, seeing, touching, etc.) Freud surmised that the illness occurred because of a conflict between the superego and the id. Failure to repress the conflict resulted in the symptoms.

When the physical symptoms occurred, there was a simultaneous lack of emotion or concern about the phenomenon, which was called *la belle indifference*. According to Freud, this lowering of the anxiety level was a primary gain, in that the anxiety, emanating from the conflict, was no longer experienced by the patient. Also, he observed that there was a secondary gain, in which the patient received side benefits from the illness. For example, when I was serving in the military service as a psychiatrist, I encountered a young Marine who had a paralyzed arm, caused by an emotional conflict. This had the secondary gain of preventing him from having to perform the routine cleaning of the barracks or any task that involved the use of his arm. The symptoms substituted for anxiety emanating from his conflict. When I removed the paralysis with an injection of sodium amytal (medical hypnosis), the anxiety resurfaced. This kind of symptom substitution is a fascinating human phenomenon.

It is noteworthy that conversion disorders are uncommon today. Many psychotherapists have never seen one case of this illness; yet, cases were very common in Freud's era. What has happened in the interim? Freud's theory was that conflicts concerning sex and aggression were the main culprits causing the neuroses. Since society has permitted the expression of aggression and sexuality to a greater degree, these disorders have diminished. But, I have seen cases of conversion disorder in uneducated, naive individuals and in families where the expression of aggressive and sensual needs are discouraged. This observation leads me to believe that Freud's theory about the origin of this form of neurosis may have some validity.

Hypochondriasis

Contrary to the popular use of the term, hypochondriasis is not simply a preoccupation with physical illness in general. Rather, it is currently defined as a fear of or a preoccupation with having a serious disease such as cancer, in spite of medical evidence that does not support such a conclusion. Persons afflicted with this disease consult with many physicians in order to confirm their suspicions about illness. Frequently, major surgery is performed at the insistence of the patient in order to cure the problem. Even after exploratory surgery proves to be negative, the patient may still believe that the cancer exists (the doctors simply were not able to find it). He or she will then go to other physicians for more opinions.

Psychotherapists have a difficult time treating this disease. Rational discussion does not dissuade the preoccupation. There are no quick and easy answers. Medication is of no real value. I have found that treating the person as a whole rather than concentrating on the claimed illness is the best approach. Sometimes, assisting the patient in dealing with his or her emotions, there is less preoccupation with the physical symptoms. Patients with this illness obsess about a serious disease instead of coping with the issues in life that would make them productive and satisfied individuals.

Somatization Disorder

Every family practitioner has a number of patients with this disorder. It is often confused with hypochondriasis, but it is more generalized and there is not the preoccupation with a serious disease. A number of symptoms (13 total) are required in various systems of the body. There are gastrointestinal, cardiac, and simulated neurological symptoms and other discomforts such as pain, or conversion symptoms explained earlier. All of the problems exist without any physical basis–at least nothing that is currently discernible by modern examination and testing. It is necessary for symptoms of this kind to exist for several years before the diagnosis can be made.

As with hypochondriasis, once the person has somatisized (displaced anxiety into physical form) his concerns to the degree mentioned, it is very difficult to reverse the process. The physician can treat the various complaints symptomatically and hope for the best. As with hypochondriasis, an attempt to treat the whole person in psychotherapy may help to reduce the physical preoccupations but will not eliminate them completely.

Pain Disorder

In this illness, the pain is present, but the physician cannot account for it by any known test or procedure. Or, if there is physical pathology, the amount of pain cannot be accounted for in relation to the degree of pathology. When there is no evident pathology that is discernible by the physician, it does not mean that there is never any source for the pain. As additional tests are invented, some new means of detecting sources of pain are discovered. For example, since the invention of the computerized axial tomography (CAT) scan, a significant number of patients with back pain due to a herniated disc have been diagnosed; these discs were not seen with traditional use of spinal myelograms. Prior to the use of CAT scans, these patients were assumed to be having pain due to a psychogenic causes.

There are a surprising number of patients who have somatoform pain disorder, with or without demonstrable pathology. I have seen patients deal with pain in stoical ways, with little or no medication. Others complain and make their pain the focus of their lives. The observer never knows what pain the patient is enduring. One thing is certain: No physician, family member, or friend should tell a person who is suffering that his or her pain is not there. "It's all in your head" is a cruel accusation. The pain is real and is felt regardless if physical pathology is present or not. My work with pain has followed two courses. When patients had the desire to come to terms with their emotional life and work out their problems, their pain almost always decreased. On the other hand, when there was neither time nor resources to pursue psychotherapy, I have found the use of pain-management tapes valuable. These are basically audio tapes that teach the patient to relax. When sufficiently relaxed, the patient is able to diminish the pain or shorten the period of time that he or she experiences it. Used repeatedly, this method can be very helpful.

DISSOCIATIVE DISORDERS

There are several syndromes that are known to the general public because of the frequency of their use as subject matter in the theatre, in films, and in novels. Who has not heard of the multiple personality

(Dr. Jekyll and Mr. Hyde)? How many novels have a protagonist with amnesia? These are engrossing themes, but actual cases are very rare in the psychotherapist's office. Having practiced psychiatry for over 30 years, I have yet to see one case of multiple personality or psychogenic fugue, in which the person suddenly leaves his or her home, assumes another identity, and has amnesia for his or her past. These syndromes are very rare indeed.

Multiple Personality

The classic case of multiple personality was depicted graphically in the film *The Three Faces of Eve.* It was derived from a true story of a patient who had three personalities. One aspect of her personality represented her more aggressive, sensual side and the other her more sedate, conservative personality. These were extremes. Eve, her third and predominant personality was a blend of the two. In Freudian terms, it was a clinical picture of the ego trying to handle the warring conflicts of the superego and the id. It made a great story, but, again, this phenomenon is rare. Recently, there has been the suggestion that persons suffering from sexual and physical abuse in childhood often develop mild cases of personality disorders. It is my opinion that much more evidence is needed before this conclusion can be validated.

A book by Flora Schreiber, *Sybil,* was based on an actual case in which the affected individual reportedly had 16 personalities. Such complicated personality structures are very hard to understand and treat. Fortunately, these problems are not an everyday experience in the lives of psychotherapists. Treatment is usually based on psychodynamic principles, often using hypnosis and occasionally medication. Because of the many personalities involved, treatment is very complicated and of long duration.

Dissociative Fugue

As explained earlier in this chapter, this condition begins very suddenly. The affected individual leaves his home without warning, assumes a new identity, and does not recall his past. There often is a conflict that precipitates the sudden departure. Hypnosis can be used to help the person recall his past. The new identity is not taken on deliberately but is done without the previous personality knowing about it. I have never seen a patient who had this fascinating but rare illness.

Dissociative Amnesia

One day, a patient of mine was out hiking with his family. He was having a good time until a severe thunderstorm occurred. He became terrified of the storm and the lack of shelter for his family. He was particularly worried about them as he was an overly conscientious father. He managed to lead his family to a sheltering overhang of rock that gave them a feeling of some security. After the storm, they completed their hike and returned home. At dinner that night, the concerned father asked his wife what had happened that day; he had no memory of the events at all.

In this form of amnesia, a significant amount of personal information is forgotten. It is not due to any organic cause and is not the kind of forgetting that is common to us all. Such amnesia may be partial, complete, of short duration, or long-lasting. Most commonly, it is of short duration. Usually, no treatment is necessary if the amnesia occurs once. However, if it is frequent, psychotherapy with or without hypnosis is indicated. This illness is not very common, but not as rare as psychogenic fugue and multiple personality.

Depersonalization Disorder

Many patients report that they have feelings of depersonalization. Without using this term, the individual will complain of feelings of detachment, of not really being present with people. The person may feel as though he is looking down on a situation or viewing it from afar. Others may complain of being in dream-like states or being in motion without much control.

While an occasional experience of this sort is not too uncommon, the diagnosis of depersonalization disorder is reserved for people who have these feelings persistently. This results in an impairment in functioning. While the feelings of depersonalization are quite real, the individual is in touch with reality and knows that the feelings he or she is experiencing are not normal.

This disorder does not occur often. Presumably, it is a reaction to some stressor. The disorder removes the person temporarily from the situation that is causing the stress. However, in time, the affected person is prevented from dealing appropriately with his environment. I have often had patients with occasional feelings of detachment, but I have never seen someone with the complete syndrome. Generally, the treatment for this condition is psychotherapy. Medication is of limited value.

WHAT CAN THE CLERGY DO ABOUT ANXIETY DISORDERS?

From the previous discussion, it should be obvious that the treatment of neuroses requires expert help. Most of the psychotherapist's work deals with the problems of people with neurotic symptoms. Even the experts are not always successful with these troubled patients. They require much patience and understanding.

The first thing that the clergy can do is have a working knowledge of these disorders. It is important that the clergy understand what a neurotic problem is and how it differs from a personality disorder. The latter is a lifelong maladaptive disorder that is going to change little over a lifetime. The clergy must handle the various personalities in their congregations as they present themselves. But, the neurotic individual may lose his phobia, depression, or anxiety and appear quite normal. The clergyperson needs to understand that the condition may be temporary. Neurotic symptoms need not go on for a lifetime.

The person suffering from neurotic symptoms may ask for nothing more than understanding and support. Your congregant may need you to listen to him or her much more than to be talked to or admonished. In short, knowing what your congregant is going through in coping with his or her neurosis and giving encouragement may be all that is necessary at any given time.

When faced with anxiety symptoms, congregants need help and encouragement in facing their fears. A patient with a phobia needs to know that avoiding the object feared is not useful in eventually conquering the phobia. Avoidance only serves to increase the fear and render the person even more helpless in coping with his or her anxiety. Someone with a fear of driving any distance needs lots of encouragement to endure the anxiety of driving farther from the security of home. Your congregant needs support as he or she copes with such symptoms. Such support from family and the clergy can be extremely important when a person is trying to overcome a phobia or any other anxiety.

The clergy can and should develop skill in recognizing the symptoms of a neurotic illness. Once having done so, it would be wise for the clergyperson to make the proper referral to a psychotherapist. If there is any question about a physical illness complicating the problem, a consultation with a physician would be in order.

If your congregant is taking a prescribed medication, he or she should be encouraged to do so on a regular basis. It has been estimated that only one-third of the advice given by doctors and therapists is followed. This includes taking medication properly.

It should be noted here that all-too-often patients cannot afford private outpatient therapy. In many communities, there are low-cost clinics that provide psychotherapy for neurotic disorders. Some are included in community mental health facilities. Others are located in community hospitals or at teaching hospitals. I am the associate director at a medical school outpatient psychiatric clinic (University of Medicine and Dentistry of New Jersey). Here, psychiatric residents, in their third and fourth year of training, treat patients, under the close supervision of senior psychiatrists. There are many such low-cost clinics throughout the country. Fees are usually based on the person's ability to pay. Major medical insurance is often of assistance in paying for this service.

Most clergy are aware of the location of clinics run by pastoral counselors in addition to clinics sponsored by religious organizations. Matching the client and the illness to the clinic or private psychotherapist is a skill that should be developed by the concerned clergyperson.

The clergy can be most effective in helping patients with anxiety disorders by recommending a prayerful attitude toward the fears and concerns that a congregant may have. Prayer may not eliminate an anxiety disorder immediately, but it will help bring the symptoms under control. It is with the combination of prayer, support from a clergyperson, and psychiatric care that the patient will have the best chance of overcoming his or her anxiety.

Chapter 8

Alcoholism and Drug Abuse

When I was a child, I looked forward to reading the Saturday comics, which had the weekly installment of the latest adventures of Buck Rogers, Flash Gordon, and others. At the top of the comic section was the picture of Shakespeare's Puck, that impish caricature of an adult, with the quotation, "What fools these mortals be!" This made a big impression on me. Indeed, we humans can be fools. Nowhere is this more obvious than in the physical and mental abuse that individuals impose on themselves with alcohol and other substances.

One day I saw a 40-year-old woman who had been drinking for many years. It was apparent that she could not benefit from office treatment, and she had to be hospitalized at a psychiatric unit of the local general hospital. She was overweight, looked ten years older then her age, and was shaking all over. She reluctantly agreed to enter the hospital. Her motivation for controlling the alcoholism was limited. On the psychiatric unit, she was detoxified, a process that takes about five to seven days, and she felt much better.

Meanwhile, during her hospital stay, she was put in contact with Alcoholics Anonymous, and she remained with AA after leaving the hospital. Thereafter, she did not require my attention at all. I credit this to the very fine work that AA does with alcoholics—more about AA later.

Such a result, although frequent, does not occur in all cases. Too often, there is a recurrence of the drinking with its many accompanying behavioral problems. I know a number of patients who have been detoxified who only succumb to the ravages of alcohol again and again after failing to take advantage of the necessary support from others in AA.

"Wine is a mocker, strong drink is raging," admonishes the Old Testament in Proverbs 20:1. Anyone who has had a bad experience with alcohol will attest to the validity of this quotation. But, there is much confusion about alcoholism, along with a great deal of denial of its existence.

WHAT IS ALCOHOLISM?

There is a cynical definition of alcoholism that is heard among those associated with the medical profession, which, unfortunately, has within its own ranks, a fairly high rate of alcohol abuse problems. "The patient is an alcoholic if he drinks more than his doctor."

Implied in this attempt at humor is that the definition of the disease is difficult to determine and that doctors have been reluctant to make the diagnosis. The classification of substance disorders is described in terms of substance dependence and substance abuse. It applies to alcohol as well as other substances. The DSM-IV carefully defines the criteria for dependence and abuse of alcohol and various drugs and refers to these as "substances." In general, the criteria are:

Substance Dependence

In order to consider someone dependent on alcohol or drugs there has to be "clinically sufficient impairment" of functioning as a result of that use. According to the DSM-IV, there also needs to be at least three or more of the following criteria to qualify as substance dependence. These behaviors must occur sometime within the period of a year.

Included in the summary are the following: a tolerance for the substance, excessive use, recurrent attempts to control substance use, and a withdrawal reaction when the substance is not regularly consumed. Further criteria are a lack of control over the substance; excessive time and effort spent in trying to acquire the substance, use it, or recover from its use; and the relinquishing of certain activities as a result of substance abuse. Finally, in spite of the fact that physical and psychological problems result, the person continues to use the substance.

Substance Abuse

The impairment resulting from abuse of substances must include one or more of the criteria listed below. As with dependence, they must be present at any time within a given year.

The substance abuse results in the person being unable to fulfill his requirements at work, home, or school. Further, he continues to abuse the substance in places where it is physically dangerous, such as driving. Substance abuse results in excessive legal problems or a series of problems with people in social or interpersonal areas as the result of substance abuse.

WHY DO PEOPLE DRINK ALCOHOL?

There is a lot of sick humor in the world of alcoholism. Individuals drink when they are unhappy, and they drink when they are celebrating. Of course, there is always an event that can make one happy or sad. Another comment often made by alcoholics is that they feel sorry for those who do not drink. The reason? Because the nondrinker, upon awaking in the morning, will never feel better the rest of the day–unlike the alcoholic, who is used to waking up with the expected hangover and then recovering. In the practice of psychiatry, I have been impressed with several reasons as to why persons drink to excess.

Early in adolescence peer pressure is of great importance. There is no denying that the need to belong to the group and to conform to the group mores often creates a powerful pressure on the young to experiment with alcohol as well as drugs.

But, what keeps one person drinking more and more as time goes on while others do not? One factor is the amount of anxiety or depression that the adolescent or young adult may have. More important, however, is the degree to which the substance, alcohol, or drug, is effective in relieving these symptoms. If there is considerable relief following ingestion of alcohol, there is good reason to continue to use that substance for the alleviation of symptoms.

In addition, some individuals appear to be able to consume copious amounts of alcohol without experiencing immediate adverse effects. That is, they do not have headaches, nausea, vomiting, excessive sedation, or other symptoms as the result of excessive alcohol intake. Their particular physiology responds differently to alcohol than in the case of most others.

In contrast, I have observed that the average person cannot drink much because he or she experiences uncomfortable side effects early, such as drowsiness, dizziness, or headaches, and consequently stops drinking. It is quite hard to become a heavy drinker when uncomfortable feelings develop with increased intake of alcohol. But, if alcohol relieves symptoms and also gives pleasant feelings of euphoria, it is not difficult to understand why it has so much appeal to some.

It appears that constitutionally some individuals are able to drink much more than others without having adverse symptoms. This is probably a hereditary trait, which may explain why some ethnic groups seem more susceptible to alcoholism than others (Kaplan and Sadock, 1988, p. 396).

There are also many rationalizations to why people drink excessively. The most common remarks are the following: "Everyone is doing it; it relaxes me," "How can I not drink when everyone at lunch in my business does it? You're expected to be one of the boys," or "I need a few drinks to get to sleep."

Our culture also contributes to the acceptability of drinking. How often have we seen the old movies in which the hassled man comes home and immediately reaches for his drink to relieve his tension. Such constant reinforcement of a habit encourages those who have a problem with alcohol to drink more.

Research may one day tell us that certain persons are prone to alcoholism because of biological factors occurring in susceptible individuals. Thus far, little has been proven in this regard, although evidence in studies of heredity tend to lead in this direction.

DRINKING PATTERNS

Alcoholics arrive at their illness along different paths. Some drink mostly at night, before, during, and after dinner. Others drink at lunch as well as the rest of the day. Many alcoholics drink in the morning as well, particularly if they experience early-morning hand and body tremors.

There are a few individuals who do most of their drinking at night, presumably to get to sleep. They may awaken during the night and drink more, and even drink again in the morning to begin the day. The patterns vary considerably, but the important thing is the amount consumed and the time over which this is done.

It is also of interest that some persons can develop serious effects of alcoholism, such as cirrhosis of the liver, after only a few years of excessive drinking. Still others can spend a lifetime drinking very heavily and not develop this disease at all.

HOW MANY PEOPLE DRINK ALCOHOL?

It is estimated that in this country about 5 to 9 million persons suffer from alcoholism. In addition, another 5 percent are heavy drinkers and have impaired functioning because of illness associated with drinking. Many lives are lost due to the disease itself or to drunken driving or other alcohol-related accidents. The extent of the problem is enormous.

In some countries, such as Italy and Japan, the incidence of alcoholism is lower. It is not clear why this difference exists. Cultural, social, and dietary differences have been cited in an attempt to explain this phenomenon, but there are no proven reasons why different groups are less prone to the disease (Kaplan and Sadock, 1988, p. 397).

TYPES OF ALCOHOLISM

There are several ways in which the disease of alcoholism manifests itself to the medical world.

Alcohol Intoxication

Alcohol intoxication is the most common form. Given enough alcohol to cause intoxication in most people, the person will display abnormal behavior. Sexual and aggressive impulses are altered, impaired judgment usually occurs, and the person is not able to perform usual tasks well. In addition, there is often slurred speech, lack of coordination, and difficulty with motor skills.

This picture is all too familiar. I am frequently astounded by the high incidence of alcohol-related problems in my practice even though my work is not primarily devoted to alcoholism. Sometimes as many as 50 percent of my patients are either themselves alcoholic or have alcoholism in their immediate family. Today, this is complicated by the increasing use of street drugs. The combined use of so-called "recreational drugs" with alcohol is especially prevalent in the young.

Alcohol Idiosyncratic Intoxication

In this form, the individual drinks a small amount of alcohol but not enough to cause intoxication in the average person. This is followed by an unusual reaction: a marked behavioral change with amnesia for the event.

The affected individual becomes very aggressive or assaultive in a way that is atypical for that person. In this condition, there seems to be a remarkable intolerance to alcohol. In some patients there has been a previous history of head injury or encephalitis. Occasionally, this abnormal reaction occurs because of the simultaneous use of tranquilizers or stimulants such as cocaine. This syndrome can be dangerous because of the violence that it engenders.

Alcohol Withdrawal Syndrome

After prolonged heavy drinking, the alcoholic may suddenly stop his or her consumption of alcohol. This usually is followed by hand tremors, nausea, vomiting, perspiration, increased heart rate, emotional irritability, and mood changes. Transitory visual hallucinations may also occur along with convulsions. Most of these symptoms disappear in about five to seven days.

Alcohol Withdrawal Syndrome with Delirium

In addition to the symptoms just described, the patient also has delirium disorientation to time and place, illusions (visual misperceptions of external stimuli), visual hallucinations, memory problems, and insomnia. This is a very dangerous illness. If untreated, about 15 percent of such patients can die. With proper treatment, the patient is usually well within a week to ten days.

Alcohol Hallucinosis

After a period of withdrawal, when the patient is not drinking, there may occur a time when he or she experiences auditory hallucinations (hears voices). Although this condition is not very common, it can last for days to months and may require hospitalization.

Alcohol Amnestic Syndrome
(Wernicke-Korsakoff's Syndrome)

When prolonged drinking occurs, there may be evidence of short-term memory loss. This may be irreversible. It is often complicated with neurological signs involving balance and eye abnormalities. The latter may be more temporary. The use of high doses of the vitamin (thiamine) sometimes ameliorates these symptoms.

Dementia Associated with Alcoholism

In this condition, there is an impairment in immediate memory as well as disorientation as to time and place. It may be present at least three weeks after a long period of drinking.

In addition to these illnesses, there are many other physical diseases associated with alcoholism, including intestinal bleeding, cirrhosis, pancreatitis, and neuropathies (nerve damage). A more recent discovery, fetal alcohol syndrome, involves the abnormalities in the newborn infant caused by mothers who drank heavily while pregnant. Doctors now advise pregnant mothers not to drink at all in order to prevent any possibility of the condition. Treatment methods for alcoholism will be discussed later in this chapter.

DRUG ABUSE

My 25-year-old patient had been taking drugs for over ten years. Beginning with adolescent drinking and cigarette smoking, she pro-

ceeded to using street drugs. She experimented with every drug
available, until it was difficult to tell what was an addiction and
what was casual use. There was no doubt about the fact that the
patient was out of control and needed hospitalization. But, even
after a short stay for detoxification, it became obvious that she
would go directly back to her drug-abusing friends and resume her
addictions. Fortunately, her family and I were able to prevail in the
recommendation that she accept rehabilitation. In this instance a
28-day stay at a hospital was sufficient, but often this is not the case.
Commonly, it is necessary for addicted individuals to be sent to
rehabilitation centers a number of times before a breakthrough
occurs.

What Is Drug Abuse?

I have always been struck by the phrase "the recreational use of
drugs." It refers to the fact that some persons take drugs on occasion to relieve symptoms, to feel less tense, or simply to get "high."
It seems to me that the term is used to rationalize drug use, so as to
make it appear less pathological. I doubt that anyone using drugs
was ever made a better person through drug use.

The criteria mentioned for the definition of alcoholism could
well be applied to define drug abuse. Although it could be refined
further, for our purposes it will suffice.

For alcoholics or the drug abusers, the main defense is denial. It
is both conscious as well as unconscious. In spite of such results as
job loss, multiple auto accidents, the revoking of a driver's license,
and the ruination of a marriage, the afflicted person still maintains that
he does not have a problem. Or, he may agree with his family and
friends that he has a disease but then proceed to continue his addiction.
Furthermore, the drug user often feels that he can control his use of
drugs. This has been referred to as the "illusion of control." It takes
drastic action to interrupt this illusion and denial and to change the
addictive patterns.

I have rarely seen an addict cure himself without considerable
outside help, although it does occur. It is well-known that a deep
religious experience can move the addict to choose a life of sobri-

ety. However, this occurs infrequently with addicts. I will discuss more on treatment and cure later.

The Frequency of Drug Abuse

One Friday after medical school classes in New York City, I ran to my apartment a few blocks away in East Harlem. I gathered up my books and laundry and headed for the subway. It was a dreary, rainy day, and I was looking forward to going to my home in the suburbs. I had on a raincoat and was carrying my old suitcase with the few belongings that I possessed. Because of the rain, I decided to run to the subway rather than walk.

Suddenly, I was aware of an old-model car keeping pace with me. One of the two men in the car jumped out and shouted at me to stop. I tried to ignore him and continued to run, but the man in the car rode on ahead to head me off as the other came from behind. My heart began to pound as I stopped. One of the men ordered me to go into the corridor of the nearest building. I was about to refuse when he showed me the gun in his shoulder holster. I needed no further persuasion. Surely, this was a mugging, or so I thought. "These guys are really going to be disappointed when they realize that I have about three dollars in my pocket and nothing of value in my suitcase." I was soon relieved, however, to learn that they were plainclothes police who were looking for drug runners. Even though I never thought that I could present an image of an antisocial character who transports drugs to acquire money, it gave me a secret pleasure to think that I could, even for a moment, appear that way. The year was 1950. Drugs, such as heroine, cocaine, marijuana, and others were more widely used in the inner cities and among certain artists and musicians.

Then came Timothy Leary with his pseudoscientific experiments with drugs; he advocated that everyone should turn off traditional thinking, and tune in to the mind-set of the counterculture, and drop-out of a traditional school program. (For a more detailed description of this era, see Chapter 2, "Parents, Society, and Heredity".) The world was affected by this pro-drug movement in a way that is known to all of us.

What has happened since 1950? After an initial marked increase in drug use, especially among young people, the pattern changed.

According to the National Institute of Drug Abuse, the use of marijuana, heroine, LSD, and other street drugs has leveled off. Since 1983, these substances have been used to about the same degree by the general public in this country. However, cocaine use has doubled, and the age at which children use drugs has lowered. I have known of adults and adolescents who started their drug use at age 9 or 10. There are reports in the literature that indicate an even lower age of onset of drug use.

I will make no attempt here to go into detail about specific drugs and their effects on the psyche and body. Rather, I would refer you to the section on general references listed in the bibliography.

Years ago, adult parents warned their children about beginning drug use, claiming that once a person starts, it leads to the increasing use of stronger and more dangerous drugs. The youth of the day argued that that was a ridiculous and illogical statement, and that parents were all wrong. Why couldn't an individual just use one drug and stop with that? The argument made some of us pause and doubt the parental worries. However, this may have been a legitimate concern. Although difficult to prove, there are probably few drug abusers who have not used at least several drugs before arriving at the end point of drug abuse. It is also doubtful that many abusers use heroine or cocaine as their first mind-altering substance.

Regarding prescription drugs, for many years drugs used by physicians to treat diseases have been controlled under the law. Certain stimulants, such as the amphetamines and Ritalin, tranquilizers such as Valium and Librium, and sedative-hypnotics such as Dalmane and Noludar have been widely prescribed. Because of easy access to these drugs, physicians and nurses have had a high degree of addiction to prescription drugs. Many patients have been given drugs by well-meaning physicians only to discover that they have a not-so-subtle addiction to their medication.

Prescription drugs have also fallen into the hands of drug dealers and have become the source of abuse for many people. These drugs, like alcohol and marijuana, have been considered by authorities as gateway drugs to the abuse of other more potent drugs.

The elderly frequently abuse drugs to relieve symptoms, or they inadvertently take more drugs than prescribed because of memory problems or failure to read or understand directions. Such abuse may lead to misdiagnosis on both a physical and mental level. The confusion and lack of alertness in the elderly is often due to over-dosage of prescribed medication.

Personality Aspects of Drug Abuse

Do certain personality types tend toward drug abuse? Perhaps. I have seen virtually all personality types involved in substance abuse. There are some qualities that are common to abusers. First of all, one has to be impressed with the compulsive nature of persons that abuse drugs or food or anything that affords pleasure. Most individuals begin abusing substances because of a sensation of pleasure or the relief of pain.

Why do some eventually become addicts and others not? This demands further research. But, there is little doubt that pleasure and the absence of pain are involved. It seems to me that symptom relief plays a large part in the onset of drug addiction.

Drug Abuse and Concomitant Psychiatric Illness

It is well-known that drug and alcohol abuse does occur more frequently in individuals with personality disorders and those who have a particular vulnerability to depression.

Often patients simultaneously suffer from drug or alcohol abuse and one specific form of psychiatric disease. For example, I have seen patients with manic-depressive (bipolar) disorder who were also alcoholics, schizophrenics who were drug abusers, and persons with eating disorders who had some form of drug abuse, as well as other disorders. This combination of mental illness and some form of chemical addiction is referred to as dual diagnosis or MICA (mental illness and chemical addiction) grouping. Some hospitals have beds set aside for patients with dual diagnoses. These patients are sometimes very difficult to treat. The treatment team has to determine which problem can be best handled first or whether the two problems can be addressed at the same time. Needless to say, these can be interesting clinical challenges.

The clergy can be very helpful with the family as well as the patient in supporting the attempt to deal with these simultaneous problems. Some individuals who stop drinking or taking drugs discover that they have a mild to moderate depression or an anxiety disorder. When the addict reaches sobriety, he or she can be treated by a psychiatrist for these disorders, just as a nonalcoholic would be treated.

TREATMENT OF ALCOHOLISM
AND DRUG ABUSE

When I took a course in sociology in college, I was asked to write a term paper on a particular person that I knew in order to illustrate what I had learned about the subject of sociology; that is, the paper was to describe the various influences in a person's life and how his or her problems evolved. The purpose of this exercise was to orient the students' thinking toward greater understanding of how individuals develop and why they behave as they do. I decided to write about my oldest brother (22 years older than I, in a family of eight children).

Without going into details about his life, it was obvious to all that he was an alcoholic. For a variety of reasons, he lived at home with us and never married. During these years, alcoholism was considered by many to be a moral problem, a case of "demon rum," and not a disease at all. The sin of drinking was handled in a way that allowed no room for understanding. And, as I later learned from AA, too much understanding in the usual empathic way could help continue the problem.

Nothing helped my brother. Family meetings at which he was exhorted to reform his aberrant ways were powerless in helping him overcome his addiction. At times he seemed to improve for a short while, but he eventually regressed further. The church elders came to visit him and counseled him on his sinful behavior, but this had no impact on his drinking. He was lonely, unhappy, and had few joys in life. He was trapped in the grip of addiction, never to be released.

My aging mother fell into the role of helping by giving him money when he was not working. The concept of codependence had not yet been discovered. He, in turn, used the money to support his drinking, and so the pattern continued. My father, who worked excessively in order to support the large family, died at age 65; he also seemed to be unable to deal with his son's alcoholism. The family felt helpless, and the church was equally unable to influence my brother in any way.

At the time, I felt that the church could have been more long-suffering rather than punitive. But, they took the established position of excommunication for the sin of alcoholism. I listened in church while the minister pronounced that my brother had committed the sin of alcoholism, and that he had not repented from his sin and reformed in spite of many admonitions. This was announced publicly three times. It was a very sad family experience.

I do not remember well what I wrote in that paper on sociology, but it led me down the road to empathy and attempts at understanding. It did not prepare me for what was to come in my professional life in appreciating the nature of addiction. Empathy and understanding are essential qualities in the psychotherapist and the clergyperson, but these traits can be grossly abused by alcoholics and drug abusers. Too easily, and with the best of intentions, we can become enablers in the addicted person's life.

Early in my practice, I encountered alcoholics who asked for tranquilizers to relieve their anxiety while they were trying to stop drinking. Frequently, they used the medication and continued their addiction. It took time for me to realize that to truly help the alcoholic, the use of medication while the alcoholic was still drinking was counterproductive. Alcoholics Anonymous realized this long before physicians, some of whom still do not accept the importance of this concept. Although there has been some mutual understanding between physicians and AA recently, many physicians remain in a state of denial regarding the nature of alcoholism.

THE IMPORTANT ROLE
OF ALCOHOLICS ANONYMOUS

I will say, flat out, that most physicians and the clergy do not have the positive effect on the alcoholic or the drug addict as the groups who work with the addictive disorders. Alcoholics Anonymous, Al-Anon, and Al-A-Teen have all been very helpful in working with alcoholics and their families. This applies equally well to other groups such as Narcotics Anonymous (NA), Drugs Anony-mous (DA), and Cocaine Anonymous (CA). I believe that the basic reason for this is very simple. Only the addicted person knows the degree to which the illness can be *denied, rationalized,* and *ignored* for so long. They are aware of all the tricks in the book. An alco-holic cannot fool a recovering alcoholic who has been in AA for some years. The support of the AA group is of enormous value. No physician or clergyperson can be available on a 24-hour basis like AA members can. And no one understands the dynamics of the alcoholic or addict like a person who has gone through the horrors and pain of alcoholism or drug addiction. AA requires honesty, confrontation with the self, and directness with others. The 12 steps of AA ask the person to look within him or herself, with the help of a Higher Power, and then to look out to others to seek amends, and go about helping those still in the grips of alcoholism. The other groups that deal with addiction basically work the same way. As far as I believe, no other program has devised a better answer.

I have seen very few alcoholics overcome their addiction without the help of AA. These cases are unusual. Some are frightened away from drinking by poor health as a result of their alcoholism, but these cases seem to be exceptions. I have seen a few respond to religious conversion experiences and give up drinking in a sudden, dramatic fashion. But for most addicted individuals, support groups are vital for their continuing sobriety.

The medical treatment of addictions is comprised of several phases. The first attack on any addiction is withdrawal from using the abused substance. In drug or alcohol withdrawal, there is always the danger of medical complications. These are usually handled best in a hospital, where any medical complication can be addressed. Some of the withdrawal effects can be deadly, as in untreated delir-ium tremens.

During the withdrawal phase, other drugs are sometimes used to relieve the symptoms of withdrawal. The physician's choice of medication varies depending on the abused substance. Following detoxification to the abused drug, a time of rehabilitation is often recommended. The purpose of this period is to provide time for education, reflection, confrontation, and coping with the massive denial that is so common to the substance abuser. AA or its equivalent is introduced at this time, and it is hoped that upon leaving the rehabilitation setting, the afflicted person will continue with this support group in his or her own community.

A drug named Antabuse has been used with some success in enabling alcoholics to refrain from drinking. When this drug has been ingested, the concomitant use of alcohol makes the patient very ill. It is hoped that this will persuade the user to refrain from drinking. I have used it in a number of patients, but I have been disappointed in the results.

SUBSTANCE ABUSE AND THE CLERGY

The degree to which the general population is affected by drugs is enormous. In this country, affluence no doubt plays a part in the extent of drug abuse. In addition, a culture that seeks immediate relief for any pain and searches for constant pleasure and stimulation is a natural environment for the abuse of drugs.

In addition to what has been said above, here are some suggestions:

1. I think that the problem facing the clergy is not unlike any other helper concerning dealing with substance abuse. Perhaps our biggest fault is in thinking that our particular area of expertise can answer all problems. I have known physicians and members of the clergy who have tried to do it all. Regardless of the problem, they did not seek help, but rather wanted to be all things to all people.

In this complicated world, we need all the help we can get. When patients ask me what I think of their reading on the subject of psychiatry or joining a self-help group or talking to their clergyperson, my response is usually, "I will take all the help I can get." Although well-informed and expert in our professions, we nevertheless are apt to be touching only one part of the elephant, as in the legend of the blind men and the elephant. Consultation with others is necessary and appropriate. I would say the same to members of the medical profession who all too often ignore the input of the clergy.

2. It is the nature of people in the helping professions to be kind and understanding. As I indicated, this may not be the best way to

assist the substance abuser. They have to be confronted often before they are able to see their denial of the problem. Understanding alone is not enough. AA has made good use of the concept of enabling, in which well-meaning helpers basically maintain the abuse through their forgiving and helpful behavior. The tendency of friends and relatives to rescue the abuser when she has fallen into trouble enables the abuser to pick herself up temporarily and continue the abuse. Those close to the abuser may need to say "no" to requests for help when she asks for money or housing. She may have to hit bottom in the abuse before the severity of her condition becomes a reality to her. For a more detailed description of these phenomena, I recommend reading the literature provided by Al-Anon on this and related subjects. I would also recommend books written for the adult children of alcoholics.

3. The clergy can be of enormous assistance in dealing with the substance abuser if they are informed on the subject and are able to confront the abuser with her disease, direct the abuser to the appropriate sources of help, and also give support to the abuser's family.

I have seen an occasional clergyperson work intensively with an addicted person in the hope of inspiring him or her to change while neglecting other routes to recovery mentioned in this book. While maximizing the value of prayer and inspiration in the life of your congregant, you can simultaneously use the other sources of help available. This way, the most can be done to ease the plight of the addicted persons among us.

Chapter 9

Organic Mental Disorders

I walked into the Intensive Care Unit of the hospital. In one of the rooms was a 28-year-old woman who had sustained a head and neck injury. While at a summer party, she carelessly dove into a swimming pool and hit her head on the bottom. The result was a spinal cord injury, as well as paralysis of her legs and possibly her arms. However, in addition to this tragic picture there were other symptoms present that were unusual.

The report from the nurse indicated that the patient was behaving strangely. She was calling out to persons not present and appeared to be seeing things. When I examined her, she was reaching out to try to change the channels on a nonexistent television set. She did this in a confused and disoriented way.

It was apparent to me that she was having visual hallucinations; however, head injuries do not generally cause such visual disturbances. Besides, the patient had just begun to have these symptoms, and it was three days since the trauma occurred. There was something strange happening.

I spoke to the patient's friend. He said that the patient had been drinking extensively at the party, but she also had been consuming large quantities of alcohol for some months preceding the accident. These were important facts.

It soon became obvious that the patient was suffering from two diseases—a severe head and neck injury and delirium tremens. The latter disease occurs when an alcoholic suddenly stops consuming alcohol after a period of heavy drinking.

The delirium tremens could be treated, and there probably would not be any permanent damage as a result, but the paraplegia would most likely remain. Two organic illnesses were present, and the mental symptoms were organic in origin.

Sometimes, mental symptoms can appear to be due to organic disease when they really originate in emotional distress. For example, panic disorders or anxiety disorders can simulate cardiac disease. Hysterical paralysis of arms or legs can appear to be a neurological problem.

Some knowledge of organic illnesses is very important to develop a full appreciation of the human mind. In a very real sense, all mental disorders are both psychological and physical, and to a greater or lesser degree, such illnesses can affect the daily ability to function. A general idea of what causes organic diseases and what is available to treat such ailments is useful to know. It is not necessary for the clergy to become expert in this area, but a knowledge of these all-too-frequently-occurring illnesses can be helpful in managing the problems that arise in dealing with them, particularly because they affect the entire family of those who are afflicted.

OVERVIEW OF ORGANIC MENTAL DISORDERS

The field of medicine has long recognized specific diseases of the mind that are primarily due to physical causes involving the brain. Mental functioning and behavior are affected variously depending on temporary or permanent interference with brain physiology. For example, alcohol ingestion can affect the brain temporarily and/or permanently, depending on the dose ingested and duration of time that the individual consumes alcohol. The same is true of other toxins that affect the mind.

If the toxic effect of a drug is brief and intermittent, there is total return of functioning to previous levels, providing the ingested dose is not excessive. If the latter occurs, permanent damage to nerve cells and destruction of nerve tissue may ensue.

The symptoms that occur from organic mental disorders may be acute, as when caused by the misfiring of nerve impulses due to external chemicals (drugs or alcohol), or the symptoms may represent more permanent physical breakdown of brain structure as in arteriosclerosis, brain tumors, or Alzheimer's disease.

In arteriosclerosis, for example, there is a narrowing of the blood vessels to the brain, resulting in decreased blood flow to brain tissue. At first this can temporarily interfere with brain metabolism and function. As the pathology increases, brain cells will die and obvious mental and physical problems will develop. Similarly, in brain tumors, the increased growth and overactivity of brain cells from a tumor causes pressure on adjacent brain tissue, resulting in symptoms related to the affected areas.

The pathology of Alzheimer's disease shows senile placques and neurofibrillary tangles in brain tissue. These are abnormalities that have replaced the normal structures in the brain. As this occurs increasingly in the frontal lobes of the brain, memory difficulties develop, followed by behavioral and cognitive disturbances. This condition develops slowly and without warning. The cause of Alzheimer's disease is as yet unknown, but many strides are being made toward uncovering the etiology.

WHAT CAUSES ORGANIC MENTAL DISORDERS?

The causes responsible for the various physical abnormalities of the brain are numerous. For the sake of simplicity, I will discuss the general factors that can cause either acute or chronic delirium and dementia (delusions, disorientation, memory defects).

A good way to remember the physical causes of these disorders is to use the mnemonic DEMENTIA (Dr. A. Yesavage, as reported by the International Medical New Service). The following list covers most of the common reasons for the etiology of these problems.

D represents drug intoxication resulting from such substances as alcohol, "street drugs," over-the-counter drugs, and drugs prescribed by physicians. The latter can include cardiac drugs, cortisone derivatives, tranquilizers, sedatives, and sleeping pills. The symptoms resulting from such intoxication varies with the type of drug and the amount ingested.

Drug interactions are another source of organic symptoms. Such interactions occur especially in the elderly, who are taking many medications simultaneously. The elderly can sometimes be confused about the proper dose and timing of the medication. When even mild memory impairments exist, the elderly often do not remember when they have taken their medication and how much to take. Drug interactions and overdosing can result.

E represents emotional disturbances. Depression in the elderly can mimic organic mental illness. Depression is usually accompanied by a slowing down of physical movements (psychomotor retardation), insomnia, mild memory impairment, and some disorientation. Depression can easily be confused with organic mental illness. It is referred to as a pseudodementia. Treatment of the underlying depression clears up the symptoms and the patient is no longer seen as demented.

The symptoms of panic disorder can resemble an adrenal tumor or hyperthyroidism. Persistent headaches may be due to stress or a brain tumor. Many other symptoms of an emotional nature can mimic organic mental disorders, and vice versa.

M represents metabolic or endocrine disorders. Such illnesses as diabetes, hypoglycemia (low blood sugar), hypothyroidism (underactive thyroid), hyperthyroidism (overactive thyroid), and pituitary tumors can cause startling symptoms of organic mental disease. These diseases can produce symptoms of depression, anxiety, and physical distress that can resemble emotional disorders. The physician must be able to distinguish one from the other. To do so, any doctor has available to him or her a wide array of laboratory tests that will assist in differentiating organic disease from nonorganic disease. But even when using every test currently available, a clinical judgment still must be made by the physician regarding the ultimate cause of the patient's distress. Mistakes are made. There are occasions when time alone can help in evaluating the true nature of a disease. In some diseases, it takes a certain amount of time before the complete syndrome becomes manifest. I have seen more than one example of this. For instance, tumors of the pancreas can often produce clinical depression as a first symptom, even before a tumor is suspected. Once the tumor is active, there are laboratory tests that will point to the diagnosis. Occasionally, a patient will consult a psychiatrist for depression, only to find out later that he has an organic illness, such as pancreatic cancer.

E is for diseases of the eyes and ears. These sense organs provide us with constant information about our surroundings, keeping us oriented and aware of what is happening in our environment. Loss of one or both of these sense organs can lead to emotional disturbances as well as prevent a person from performing cognitive tasks well. A deaf elderly person can become mildly paranoid due to hearing deficits. People who have become blind may feel that they are the object of pity. Until we experience a loss of hearing or sight, there is little awareness of the moment to moment dependence on these senses for our daily existence.

N is for nutritional disturbances. At one time, many individuals suffered from vitamin deficiencies, especially the water-soluble vitamins (B-complex and C). Such illnesses as beriberi and pellagra, due to inadequate B-complex vitamins, are not generally seen in developed countries where nutritional standards are high. The same is true for scurvy, which is caused by vitamin C deficiency.

Poor nutrition is prevalent among the elderly, the homeless population, alcoholics, patients with severe diarrhea, and those with a variety of other medical conditions. Usually, these nutritional deficiencies are easily detected and corrected. When first seen, however, a number of patients with one of these illnesses may appear to have organic brain dysfunction.

T represents trauma and tumors. Frequently, an alcoholic or an elderly person can sustain a head injury and not recall its occurrence. Yet, the trauma can be responsible for the presenting symptoms. Usually, there is a clear-cut history of trauma or physical evidence of injury, which must be evaluated in terms of mental functioning.

Brain tumors present special problems for the psychotherapist. A tumor can be silent and not show symptoms at the beginning of therapy. It is a therapeutic nightmare to treat a patient's depression with psychotherapy and medication, only to discover later that she is suffering from a brain tumor. A host of tumors can cause depression, particularly those affecting the frontal lobes. Some are slow growing (meningiomas), and others grow rapidly and can cause death quickly (glioblastomas).

Fortunately, there have been great strides made in diagnosing brain pathology. New techniques such as the CAT scan and magnetic resonance imaging (MRI) have been developed to assist the physician in accurately diagnosing brain pathology. More discussion about these new techniques will follow.

I includes any kind of infection, such as encephalitis, meningitis, and brain abscess. Such pathology can be caused by bacteria, viruses, or other organisms. Infections that occur in the heart, as in endocarditis, can send tissue emboli from the heart to the brain. Patients with chronic bronchitis or emphysema can suffer from a low oxygen level in the brain, which can result in confusion and disorientation.

A is for arteriosclerosis. In this condition, as mentioned, the blood vessels narrow and blood flow to the brain is decreased resulting in confusion, disorientation, and memory loss. If prolonged, personality changes can also occur.

DIAGNOSING ORGANIC BRAIN DISEASE

In attempting to diagnose these diseases, it is first necessary to obtain from the patient and family a good medical history. Metabolic illnesses, nutritional deficiencies, infections, and drug abuse can be documented using careful questioning.

Laboratory tests are very helpful in establishing the existence of these diseases. The spinal tap is still used widely in diagnosis. Spinal fluid pressure, the chemical contents of the fluid, and the presence of blood in the spinal column or infection can all reveal various pathology. Perhaps the most important breakthrough in the diagnosis of organic mental illness is the invention of new radiologic techniques.

The use of the traditional X ray to visualize abnormalities of the brain was very limited. Subsequent procedures have increasingly refined the ability of the physician to uncover specific brain pathology. The pneumoencephalogram was used extensively at one time to diagnose certain space-occupying lesions such as tumors or abscesses. In this procedure, air is injected into the spinal column. It is allowed to fill the spaces in the brain normally containing cerebral spinal fluid. Any changes in the appearance of these spaces as seen on an X ray would be suggestive of pathology. This technique was very limited in its usefulness compared to the more modern methods.

For a period of time the brain scan was used to further help define areas of pathology. In this procedure a radioactive substance is injected into the patient's bloodstream. When it reaches the brain, X rays are taken. If the normal blood vessels are distorted, brain abnormalities are suspected. This technique was useful but quite limited because it could only detect large abnormalities. When the CAT scan was invented, great progress occurred in the diagnosis of organic brain disorders.

The CAT scan is able to produce a series of pictures of pathology present at any level of the brain. Knowing the normal brain structure based on large-scale studies, radiologists can observe abnormal findings. The technique refined what could be observed in the soft tissue of the brain so that even minute changes in form and structure could be noted.

Soon to follow was the nuclear magnetic resonance (NMR) scanning, or magnetic resonance imaging (MRI). In this procedure, a radio signal is applied to the brain in a uniform magnetic field. While the polarity of the magnetic field is changed, the brain may be viewed in many planes and directions on a computer monitor. The composite findings of such a procedure result in even further delineation of brain pathology. For example, the minute unraveling of the covering (myelin sheath) of a nerve fiber was observed for the first time in a live person. Such findings are present in patients with multiple sclerosis. Prior to the use of the MRI, the diagnosis could only be verified at the time of autopsy.

Both the CAT scan and the MRI are available in most community hospitals or nearby medical centers. These newer radiologic systems have greatly increased the physician's ability to diagnose organic brain disease.

As more and more is discovered about the nature of these illnesses, it becomes increasingly important that an early diagnosis be made. Prompt treatment for diseases such as brain tumors can lead to more favorable prognoses.

The latest innovation in radiological imaging is the positron emission tomography (PET) scan. At present this is a research tool and is not generally used in hospitals to diagnose brain dysfunction. A simpler version of this technique is called single photon emission computed tomography (SPECT).

While the CAT and MRI scans measure the form and structure of the brain, the PET scan is capable of discerning brain function (i.e., metabolism rather than form). In this procedure, glucose is labeled with a positron-emitting isotope (fluorine 19). It is injected into the bloodstream. When the PET scanner views the brain along various axes, the parts of the brain metabolizing glucose can be observed by the changes in colors seen on a computer monitor. Permanent photographs of what is seen on the monitor can be taken at any level. Thus, the specific areas of glucose metabolism can be determined. Similar studies can be done with other substances such as amino acids and drugs. The site of action of a metabolite or drug can be determined with a high degree of specificity. Disease is suspected in locations that have altered metabolism.

PET scan research will provide much information about possible causes of diseases and will be very helpful in determining treatment. The researchers have only begun to tap the knowledge that will eventually be available from PET scan studies. Prior to the invention of the PET scan, relatively little was known about brain function. Now, new information is being obtained with unusual speed.

As I have noted, many organic brain disorders can cause emotional stress. Research is being done now examining the relationship of stress to the immune system. Such inquiry studies the individual's reaction to diseases ranging from infection to cancer. An example of this is the work done by Dr. Marvin Stein of the Mt. Sinai School of Medicine at the City University of New York and Steven J. Schleifer and Steven E. Keller of the University of Medicine and Dentistry of New Jersey. Their studies reveal that clinical depression suppresses the immune system, and the relief of depression restores the immune system to its normal state. It is believed that stress influences the immune system adversely, and that such stress can be instrumental in laying the groundwork for certain physical diseases.

ORGANIC DISEASE MASQUERADING AS EMOTIONAL ILLNESS

In the field of counseling, one must always be aware that many physical illnesses do have emotional aspects and that primary stress-related ailments have physical components.

Likewise, physical disease can exist with little emotional reaction, and severe mental illness can occur with little effect on bodily functions. There is a tendency among psychotherapists to view every problem that a person presents as being psychologically based. The therapist must be aware and cautious to rule out physical causes of emotional illness.

The following are two case histories of patients who were seen in psychotherapy for what appeared, at first, to be emotional disorders; they later developed organic mental illness. These cases are presented to alert the clergy, who may be counseling, that such organic illness can be causing emotional symptoms, or at least can be contributory to the patient's illness. Obviously, any individual can have both an emotional and an organic illness simultaneously, or one may follow the other.

Case 1: Roger

One day I examined a 50-year-old man named Roger in my office; he had the following complaints. He was depressed and was convinced that his wife was having an affair with another man, which his wife denied. His suspicion and jealousy were mild, as was his depression.

After the initial interview, I elected to treat Roger with psychotherapy and an antidepressant. Since Roger had had a depression several years prior to this second episode, it made sense to treat him in this fashion.

After two months, Roger showed no improvement. I admitted him to the hospital. Roger's internist did some screening tests and discovered that he had an elevated sedimentation rate. This indicates an inflammatory process in the body that is not specific for any one disease. Roger became increasingly confused and had severe loss of recent memory. His behavior grew worse, and he required nursing care around-the-clock.

An MRI of the brain was done, and it showed evidence of an inflammatory process in the blood vessels of the brain (vasculitis). Roger was treated with anti-inflammatory medication as well as major tranquilizers to control his behavior. Although he improved temporarily, his condition deteriorated and grew increasingly organic.

Case 2: Lily

A 69-year-old woman named Lily was referred to me for treatment of depression. It was two years after her husband died. She was clearly depressed, was socializing poorly, and had physically slowed down. Lily's appetite had declined, and she was sleeping poorly. These were all symptoms of major depressive disorder.

After a course of antidepressants and supportive psychotherapy, Lily's general condition improved, but she never reached her previous level of functioning. I noticed that on occasions, perhaps several times in a session, she would make unusual errors in speech. For example, she said, "This week I took a foot stepward"–instead of a step forward. I noted these abnormalities and suspected early organic disease. A neurological examination and CAT scan were negative.

Treatment was continued on a monthly basis to follow her course. More verbal errors occurred although the patient's mood was normal. Within a year, it became obvious that Lily was suffering from early Alzheimer's disease, and this was confirmed by a repeat CAT scan.

WHAT CAN THE CLERGY DO?

In the two examples cited, what appeared to be common psychological symptoms was later diagnosed as early (prodromal) symptoms of an organic disease. Quite possibly, both an emotional and physical illness were present simultaneously. In both cases, it would have been impossible to diagnose the organic disease when the patients were first seen. Recognizing the subtle changes in symptoms can often provide clues to the possibility of underlying organic pathology.

One would not expect a member of the clergy to recognize the significance of such subtle changes. However, it would be inappropriate to assume that changes in behavior are always due to the obvious presenting psychological problems. Physical disease in the brain can cause a host of behavioral and psychological changes, and anyone in a counseling role should be aware that such phenomena are possible.

If in doubt, the clergyperson, as a counselor, should obtain medical confirmation that organic illness is not present. This should be repeated if there is any doubt concerning the nature of new symptoms that arise during the period of counseling.

Persons with organic disorders need much support. Depending on the condition, their level of functioning can be variously compromised, especially in chronic illnesses. The clergy can assist in the person's adjustment to having caregivers at home or to hospital or nursing home care. If a clergyperson has a solid relationship with a congregant, he or she may be able to foster a smoother transition in the changing health care needs of the affected individual. Often the family is too emotionally involved with the sick person to help effectively. The clergy can play an effective role in helping communication between the various caregivers and the congregant through supporting the goals that these caregivers request.

There is often much guilt within a family when illness occurs. Objectively valid guilt can be handled by clergy in an appropriate religious manner, while neurotic guilt must be recognized as such and, if severe enough, the family member should be referred to a psychotherapist for treatment.

The positive and negative personality traits that an individual has are usually exaggerated in organic illnesses, especially in the elderly. It is important for the clergy to keep this in mind when advising the family about a sick member. A degree of tolerance for excesses of behavior along with firm boundaries for what is acceptable behavior is the best guideline to offer the family.

It has been said that a human being is an adult once and a child twice. This is sadly true in the case of senility. When a parent reaches old age and becomes helpless and dependent, the adult children of the elderly person often continue to behave with him or her as though the old parent-child dyad still existed. That is, when the elderly, debilitated person is unreasonable or excessively demanding and angry, the adult child often has trouble being firm and assertive. It is important to take control. When the adult child assumes the parental role instead of the child role, the entire relationship changes. I tell such adults that the parent is behaving like a child and therefore has to be treated like a child. As changes are made in the relationship, the elderly person gradually accepts the new role and becomes more relaxed and secure. A clergyperson can be very helpful in bringing about this reversal of roles.

Chapter 10

Personality Disorders

The clergy and physicians have something in common—problem people. When dealing with relatively normal and healthy personalities, our work is uncomplicated and rewarding. But, when faced with difficult personalities, our various jobs become problematic.

Individuals with personality disorders can make life very trying at times, and even intolerable. You can feel ready to quit your work as clergyperson, fantasize about other professions, or just want to get away from it all.

Some time ago, I was treating a young man who was having trouble with interpersonal relationships at his job. When I got to know him well, and felt that I had a good understanding of his problem, I ventured to suggest that he might try a different approach to people. This was the beginning of a series of suggestions that I rendered, all of which he immediately rejected. Either he had tried it before or he devalued the content of my suggestion.

Such an interaction is quite frustrating. Thoughts came to me, such as, "What does this man want from me? Everything that I mention is no good. He knows it all; yet, he is asking for help. One of these days I am going to. . ." It dawned on me, finally, that this was a countertransference situation that needed to be confronted. (For more on the phenomenon of countertransference, see Chapter 15, "Pastoral Ethics: A Psychiatrist's View.") I told my patient, in a more delicate way, what I had been thinking: "I am puzzled by the fact that most everything that I have suggested to you has been unsatisfactory and of no use to you. It appears to me that you have difficulty accepting advice from me."

He was not surprised; I had caught him at his game, about which he was partially aware. In fact, a look of recognition came to his face, because he had been told this before by friends and relatives. He admitted that this was a fault that had been with him as long as he could remember; he had trouble controlling it. We were able to talk about this negative aspect of his personality. I identified his basic passive-resistant personality and documented its existence from his past history. Only then did therapy move forward along a much more productive path. As one might expect, this phenomenon repeated itself on occasions throughout the course of the therapy.

What are personality disorders? The glossary of the DSM-IV defines these disorders as "deeply ingrained, inflexible, maladaptive patterns of relating, perceiving, and thinking, of sufficient severity to cause either impairment in functioning or distress." Psychiatrists describe this as ego syntonic; that is, the affected individual is not particularly bothered by the defect. Rather, he bothers others. In contrast, the neurotic person is ego dystonic, meaning that he is made considerably upset and symptomatic by his condition. Also, to be diagnosed with a personality disorder, the individual must be 18 years of age or older. Before this age, specific forms of behavioral styles are called traits, rather than disorders. For example, a child who frequently misbehaves, as judged by general standards of society, does not necessarily grow up to have an antisocial personality disorder. Although he may show antisocial traits in childhood, these may disappear before adulthood.

How do personality disorders differ from a neurosis? The latter is characterized by a conflict that produces symptoms, which can manifest at any time of life and may disappear gradually or abruptly. Personality disorders are enduring and usually lifelong, although there is a tendency for personality characteristics to modify somewhat with aging.

A person with an obsessive-compulsive personality disorder is excessively orderly, neat clean, and unduly concerned about time and possessions. These are lifelong personality traits. In contrast, the person with the neurotic illness, obsessive-compulsive disorder, may suddenly begin to obsessively hand-wash, which must be carried out in a ritualistic way or else the patient will encounter severe anxiety. Such symptoms can resolve with treatment, or sometimes symptoms resolve spontaneously.

Being able to determine the various personality styles or personality disorders in particular can be very rewarding in the therapeutic process as well as in the life of the clergyman with his congregants. I would like to describe some of the more troublesome personality disorders, but, before doing so, it is important to discuss the latest findings in the development of the personality.

HOW DOES THE PERSONALITY DEVELOP?

As discussed in Chapter 2, "Parents, Society, and Heredity," a child is not born with a *tabula rasa*, upon which a personality is constructed. Rather, there are hereditary factors that play a significant part in his or her development.

Some years ago, an interesting study was done in New York by Thomas and Chess. Their results are published in a book titled *Temperament and Development.* They observed normal newborn infants in the nursery on a daily basis and they continued to observe these children on a weekly basis, and periodically thereafter at their homes. The study continued for 20 years. The results were fascinating. It revealed several kinds of temperament, upon which the personality is presumably constructed during the period of growth and development.

Temperament was defined as behavioral style. Approximately 65 percent of the children had one of three types of behavioral styles. The first to be observed was the loud, crying infant, who slept little, was seldom quiet, but who made his presence known to all. As this type was studied over the years, he remained basically the same. This group was called the Difficult Child and comprised 10 percent of the study.

A second type was the quiet child, who slept a lot, was not demanding, and cried only when he or she was hungry or had a physical need (hot, cold, need to be changed, etc.). This group was labeled the Easy Child and was observed in 40 percent.

The third behavioral style to evolve in this study was called the Slow-To-Warm-Up Child (15 percent). Everyone is familiar with this category. This is the child who enters new situations with caution. If the child is new in the neighborhood, he would not approach other children and ask to play with them, as would a more aggressive child. Fearing rejection, or perhaps just being more cautious by nature, he will stand around and observe until he is asked to play. Or, when a ball comes his way he may be helpful and return it to the others. Eventually, he is asked to join the game, and then he feels comfortable. This child "warms up slowly."

All three types of behavioral styles developed personalities that tended to maintain the characteristics that they displayed in infancy in their basic temperaments. Even 20 years later, these traits endured. The few exceptions to this were in situations where gross psychological problems occurred that caused a change in behavioral style. However, these changes were usually temporary.

Did anything else change or modify the traits? Yes. The authors of the study observed that there were some factors that made a difference. The personalities of the parents may play a role. For example, if a quiet child grows up in a family in which the parents are very active, the interaction could present a problem. Very busy parents have trouble understanding a child who does not need a lot of friends, who prefers to sit and read, and who does not think that running around and making noise is much fun. This mix of parental and child personality traits can cause difficulties in childrearing and lead to a neurotic interaction, but the child's basic temperament will remain much the same. The quiet child will seldom become an aggressive adult. Likewise, the aggressive individual does not in adult life become quiet and reserved, unless she encounters severe emotional stress.

The results of this study placed a new light on personality theory. Since the time of Freud, most of us working in the mental health field assumed that the parents were almost solely responsible for the outcome of a child's personality. As Thomas and Chess state in their book,

> As mental health professionals we became increasingly concerned at the dominant professional ideology of the time, in which the causation of all child psychopathology, from simple behavior problems to juvenile delinquency to schizophrenia itself, was laid at the door of the mother. (p. 5)

The real value of such a study is that it is prospective, that is, the outcome is observed over time. In the past, most psychological studies have been retrospective, that is, based on clinical case reports, in which the adult remembers what he or she experienced, and psychological theories are advanced on the basis of such information. It is known that the patient's memories about his or her past are often grossly inaccurate, but it is assumed that the feelings that the individual has about past experiences are the important ingredient. There is little doubt that in the work of psychotherapy, feelings are very important. But, psychological theories may not rest very securely on such information and are subject to a variety of interpretations, hence, the disparate schools of psychoanalysis.

Other recent studies of identical twins who were reared apart reveal that there is a strong hereditary correlation in personality traits in the areas of aggressiveness and emotionality.

It appears that there are traits that are inborn and perhaps dependent on the gene pool. As a child develops, however, he or she learns to trust or distrust, depend on others normally or become too dependent, etc. But, in the long run, his or her basic temperament will remain much the same. This is an important observation to keep in mind both in the mental health field and in education. It is also very significant in dealing with congregants, as any member of the clergy can attest. You cannot change an individual's temperament although you may be able to modify the behavior. A recent convert to a particular faith may change behavior drastically for the better, but his or her basic temperament in dealing with life and interactions with people will remain much the same.

CLASSIFICATION OF PERSONALITY DISORDERS

There are 11 personality disorders listed in the DSM-IV. I will briefly define them and then discuss the disorders that are the most difficult to handle for the clergy and other helpers. As you read through these types, perhaps you will recognize in them some of your most troublesome congregants.

1. The *paranoid personality* is lacking in basic trust, always expecting others to do her harm. She suspects hidden motives in the actions of others; she becomes angry and jealous easily and does not forgive gracefully. She is suspicious and doubtful and does not make friends easily.

2. The *schizoid personality* is withdrawn, aloof, and cold, has poor interpersonal relationships, and is mildly autistic (given to much lonely preoccupation and daydreaming).

3. The *schizotypal personality* has an excessive belief in magical thinking. This personality is very superstitious and claims to have a sixth sense—to be clairvoyant and telepathic. He will tell you that he is psychic, and can feel the presence of deceased persons in the room with him. He has few close friends; his affect (feeling tone) is often inappropriate to the content of the particular conversation. He may appear odd and eccentric.

4. The *antisocial personality* has a history of poor school performance, truancy, stealing, and early sexual behavior that is inappropriate to his age group. He may be overly aggressive, cruel to animals, and involved in more fighting than others. In general, he had a behavior problem in childhood. As an adult he performs poorly and does not conform to social norms. He often accumulates debts, continues to steal, and seldom tells the truth. He is not responsible regarding work, is impulsive, and appears to have little ability to learn from his past experiences. He is capable of cold-blooded crimes, about which he has no remorse.

5. The *borderline personality* is one who tends to see others in black-or-white terms, either the best or the worst. She is emotionally very unstable and can be feeling fine in the morning and suicidal at night, only to feel well again the next day. She has identity concerns, and often is confused about her sexuality. On occasion "mini-psychotic" episodes may be present for several days, with or without hospitalization. Maintaining friendships is difficult for this personality. Her impulsiveness may involve sexual excesses, substance abuse problems, or other deviant behavior.

6. The *histrionic personality* is one who loves attention and tends to think in terms of extremes. More often female than male, this person expresses herself in exaggerated terms. The histrionic person is constantly looking for approval and praise, is frequently seductive, tends toward immediate gratification of needs, and is emotionally shallow. She is excessively concerned with physical appearance. While delightful to be around for a short time, she does not sustain positive relationships with others over time, resulting in difficult interpersonal relationships.

7. The *narcissistic personality* is the truly selfish person. He possesses grandiose ideas about himself, a sense of entitlement, and an extreme sensitivity to the criticism of others. He takes advantage of others for his own benefit, and he expects to be noticed even without accomplishing anything special. He has fantasies of great success and wants to be admired and adored while being envious of others. At the same time, he has little sympathy for others and appears incapable of having feeling for others.

8. The *avoidant personality* is the individual who is fearful of social situations. She is shy and fears criticism of others. As a result, she has few friends, and seldom ventures an opinion in public for fear of being ridiculed. There is also a fear of being embarrassed in public by showing signs of anxiety in a physical form such as crying or blushing. As the name implies, there is an avoidance of any implied threat in social relationships.

9. The *dependent personality* is one who relies excessively on others. He is fearful of being wrong, hates criticism, and as a result, is afraid to make decisions. This person does not like to be alone, has problems of self-assertion, and fears rejection.

10. The *obsessive-compulsive personality* is the person who tends to be the perfectionist. Neat and orderly, she usually goes beyond what is necessary in working on a task, often making it impossible to complete the task. She is excessively concerned with details, standards, and appearances, and has problems working with others because they do not meet her requirements. She may be a workaholic, overly scrupulous, and given to miserliness. This type of personality has a particular difficulty expressing feelings and appears to be very cold emotionally.

11. *Disorder not elsewhere classified* is the category that is used when these personality types do not fit the particular individual being considered. Some persons have a combination of traits of different personalities, and hence cannot fit neatly into any of the defined categories.

There is another personality type that was included in the DSM-III-R, which was deleted from the new classification. It is being studied further, but most people in the mental health field have accepted the presence of the passive-aggressive personality. He is easy to recognize; he is the person who has the appearance of conforming to others while dragging his feet emotionally. He resists doing what is asked of him, or consents to do so and then procrastinates doing it. He agrees to take on a job and then has to be reminded that things are due. He seldom finishes a job and has many excuses for failing to complete the required work. At other times he resists the demands of others and becomes irritable or angry. Some individuals in this group are constantly aggressive and act aggressively on all occasions, even when it is inappropriate.

Most people will not fit these classifications very well. If some of the above mentioned traits predominate in a person, however, he may be a particular problem to the clergyperson or the psychotherapist. Trying to understand the behavior of these various personality types can be very useful in pastoral work.

PERSONALITY TYPES THAT GIVE YOU PROBLEMS

As a clergyperson, you will at some time encounter all of the above personality types. In the practice of psychiatry, I certainly have met them all. One of the difficulties in dealing with these individuals is that we as helpers often have the naive idea that if we only treat these people nicely, think well of them, provide enough love and affection toward them, pray for them, and trust them, all will be well. Too often this approach does not work. It is my contention that if you understand the nature of these personalities and work within the framework of their limitations, you can avoid a great deal of frustration and pain in your pastoral role.

Example 1

The first person to consider is the woman who is expecting something tragic to happen although there is no overt evidence for it. The reaction is one of hysteria. She calls you in a panic and must see you immediately. You accommodate her and see her that afternoon. As she approaches, you are aware that there are others accompanying her. Yes, her mother, grandmother, and husband are all there to support her. She is crying hysterically, and very fearful that she may have cancer. No physician has made a diagnosis. Nothing has been confirmed.

What would be the best way to find out what is going on? What should you do with the other family members? How do you best quiet the hysterical (histrionic) concerns of this congregant?

Individuals who become hysterical tend to remain so when there is a crowd around them, much like the child who is having a temper tantrum. This does not occur by any process of thought or design on the part of the affected person. It just happens as a result of his or her personality, and is the typical reaction pattern displayed toward a variety of stressors. Given a histrionic personality, the pattern cannot be changed easily, but it can be handled in a way that reduces anxiety quickly and facilitates improved behavior.

The first rule of thumb is to talk to the person *alone,* while the family remains in another room. Talking to the disturbed hysterical person alone cannot be stressed enough. This almost immediately reduces the overreaction to the perceived harm. A soft voice is very soothing to such a person, and a few questions regarding the anticipated problem will further calm things. Quiet reassurance will continue the process, and after perhaps one-half hour, the individual will be measurably calmer. At this point, I would invite *one* family member into the room to review the situation and gather further details about the problem. After examining the issues, perhaps a few suggestions would be appropriate. But, the most important aspect to recognize about this example is the process that is most effective in dealing with the hysterical person. For other personality disorders, this process might not work well at all.

To continue helping, you should phone your congregant a few hours later to see how he or she is doing. Such personal concern and follow-through has enormous reassuring value to such a person. Furthermore, if you have any specific advice, it is a good policy to write it down because hysterical persons tend to be so distraught that they soon forget what you have told them.

The basic idea is that you cannot change the personality of your congregants, but you can work with them in ways that are consistent with their particular personality traits.

Example 2

One of your hardest workers tells you that he has some suggestions to help you with the congregation. But, he is asking to talk to you at a time that is inconvenient to you. Yet, you do not want to ignore him because you know from previous experience that he is a very neat, careful, punctual, obsessive individual.

What should you do about your well-planned agenda that day? How do you fit him into it? What are you going to do when he suggests, in great detail, and at great length, a major overhaul of everything in your congregation? In short, how does one deal with the obsessive personality who demands immediate time and attention?

Knowing that the concept of time is of great importance to such a person, I would explain to him that I cannot discuss such an important matter in a short amount of time, but I can make an appointment to talk about it at a mutually agreed upon hour. This will appeal to his sense of orderliness–everything in its *time* and *place*. But, when you get to see him at the scheduled time, he is apt to pull out a list of 30 suggestions that you are supposed to try. He has given much thought to the matter and will not be dismissed lightly. What can you do? My suggestion is that you look over the list and take note of the ideas without discussing them. Tell him that you appreciate the fact that he has spent so much *time* on these matters and that you would like to keep the list to consider the ideas carefully when you have more *time*. Then ask which two or three of the 30 items are of greatest concern. Select these for discussion for the time that is currently available.

This scenario recognizes the concerns about time and detail that the obsessive person has. Given his expressed interest, it is important that he be involved in some way in the work of the congregation. Of course, the best work to give him is the type that involves detail, which can be worked on alone–because only he can "do it right." If one of the ideas is useful to you, he will also enjoy the proper recognition when thanked by you. A job well done is especially important to the obsessive individual. As with other personality traits, your congregants will respond best when you use their personalities in the service of your helping.

Example 3

You will recognize this personality. She is generally quite agreeable. When you ask for help, she is perfectly willing to volunteer, but that is as far as it goes. Weeks later, you realize that the job was not done. At first it is hard to understand. She seemed so eager to do the task. What happened?

Psychiatrists call this person the passive obstructionist. She is at one end of the passive-aggressive scale. While superficially co-operative, she will "yes" you to death and then procrastinate, since this is her main problem. She consciously wants to be helpful and participate, but unconsciously, she is still playing the game that she never stopped playing with her parents: "Take out the garbage, dear." "Yes, mother." But, it never gets done.

The passive obstructionist is a well-meaning person who aspires to great heights. Usually, she is a perfectionist at heart. In her opinion, she really must do something spectacular or it is not worth doing. I once saw such a person, a college student who was asked to write a biography of an historical figure. Instead of choosing a well-known person, on whom there would be considerable material, he chose an obscure eighteenth-century political character. After consulting with three major libraries, finding little data, and wasting considerable time, he had to abandon his project for lack of sufficient material, thus succeeding in failing yet another course. His passive-aggressive personality again prevented him from succeeding.

Once you discover that you are dealing with this kind of personality in one of your congregants, you have to adapt different strategies. First of all, she does not do well with long-term projects. Give this person short-range goals, specify a time limit, and call the day before you expect it to be ready. In suggesting this method, you will recognize that you are not attempting to change the personality, but merely working within the framework of the possible for that person.

You might consider giving her things to do that are even more immediate, such as ushering, collecting things, handing out material at a service, etc. Of course, she may be late for duty and not show up on time, but she probably will be there. After all, nobody is perfect!

Example 4

At the other end of the passive-aggressive scale is the aggressive personality. One Saturday afternoon I walked into a crowded department store. The men's clothing section had about 30 to 40 customers milling around. There were only three salesmen. It looked as though it would take considerable time to have a salesperson assist me. In walked a very short, stocky man. He assessed the situation and immediately bellowed, "Where the hell is the help around here, anyway?" He was so loud that everyone in that section turned to see who was yelling. He got immediate service. As typically happens, the aggressive personality gets what he wants quickly, although irritating many in the process. How do you deal with the aggressive personality in your congregation? With difficulty!

This kind of personality *is* difficult to deal with, but he sometimes can be good at getting others to do things; he generally moves fast and is impatient with those who are passive. His unconscious modus operandi is, "The best defense is a good offense!" This dictum is learned early in life. Perhaps it is to some extent inherited. The aggressive person often cannot help being this way; he comes on strong without even trying.

It may seem odd, but if you are aggressive with such a person, he often becomes more congenial. It is as though he then understands you or prefers you that way. Better still, if you meet him with an aggressive remark before he hits you with one, he appears to respond better. Tiptoeing around the aggressive person does not make him less aggressive. Rather, he seems to enjoy the fact that others are afraid or at least intimidated by him.

So, do *not* "try a little tenderness"; try a little aggression. It may be the best way that you can show love toward him. Your usual kind and gentle manner may not work well with the aggressive personality. A change in your style may help you handle him better.

Example 5

The borderline personality is probably the most difficult person to handle in a group. One of the main traits that such a personality shows is the tendency to stress the importance of something one day only to deny the significance of it the next day. If you remember what was said the day before and base your actions on it, you may be astounded by such sudden changes. Let me illustrate.

One night I was called to see a patient at her home because she had taken an excess of sleeping pills in an apparent suicide attempt.

When I arrived, it was obvious that the amount of medication that she had taken was not dangerous. After much discussion, I decided that she could be safely left in her husband's care. I made an appointment to see her in my office early the next morning. When she arrived, I asked her how she felt. Was she still depressed and suicidal? She looked at me with a quizzical and puzzled expression, as though she had no idea what I was talking about. She denied any suicidal thoughts and minimized the events of the night before, as though they were about as important as a television program she had watched. Her thoughts were now on a different plane while mine were still on the previous evening.

Another frustrating behavior of the borderline personality is his tendency to either aggrandize others or consider them to be devils. The use of adverbs in speech that qualify or moderate concepts or describe people does not seem to be a part of his vocabulary.

Somewhat related to this is the most distressing trait in this personality—the ability he has to "split" groups. He has an uncanny knack of taking sides in a group and alienating one side from the other. Peacemaking is not part of his agenda. He only feels secure in a tight group with a common enemy. This is somewhat reminiscent of the cliques that form in junior high and high school. The leaders of these groups are occasionally skilled borderline personalities. If you are striving toward a sense of community in your congregation, the individual with a borderline personality will see to it that you are frustrated to the point of wanting to quit the clergy and pursue another field.

How does one deal with this personality type? There is no magical answer. It requires considerable patience and consistency. Without ignoring his excesses, you should not take everything that he says as being meant seriously. Tomorrow he will have a different opinion, spoken with as much conviction as the day before. Today's charitable cause may be past history and unimportant tomorrow. The mere fact that you identify such a personality disorder as having certain features will remove you somewhat from the emotional content of the interaction. Try then to understand the nature of such a person, who is so insecure as to find it necessary to have such disturbing defenses.

The other danger that this individual displays is the tendency to envision you as a hero, to see you as the *best* clergyperson that ever lived, only to discover that you, too, have feet of clay. Be on guard when you are too much admired by a congregant. It probably will not last. You may be in for a big fall in his eyes, particularly if you are unsuspecting of the event. Sooner or later the borderline personality will discover your faults and bring them to the attention of other congregants.

Furthermore, the borderline personality is not very stable and tends to be impulsive. Although initially appealing and even seductive, he is not known for follow-through. You would not want to give him a lot of responsibility, especially individual responsibility.

Example 6

Then there is the "doubting Thomas." There is at least one in every congregation. I am not speaking here of her theology, but of her nature. She doubts everything, except what she can verify. This person strongly suspects that everyone is out to get her; thus, she has to be on guard at all times. Since she has difficulty trusting, it is doubtful that she will confide in you. This represents a paranoid personality, which should not to be confused with paranoid schizophrenia. The former is a long-standing series of personality traits, while the latter is a serious mental illness that develops in adolescence or in young adult life. (See Chapter 5, "Schizophrenic Disorders".)

With this individual, it does not make much sense to spend a lot of time trying to convince her of things. It matters little how logical you are; she will not budge. Even when it comes to factual matters, she is not influenced by what you can show her in a book. Rather than appeal to logic in religious concerns, it is better to rely on faith.

If this kind of personality asks you to prove that God exists, do not play the game. She will have plenty of arguments to cast doubt on everything you say. If the person has personal problems with other congregants, you cannot prove that others meant no harm in saying something that she regards as personally meant for her.

The best way I know to approach a person with a paranoid personality is to be frank and firm. Your usual kind and gentle approach will not work well. Try asking the question, "How do you expect others to be friendly with you when you never believe them? You will always have problems with people until you begin to trust them."

I have told medical students that if such a person could not accept the fact that she needed an emergency operation after the usual medical explanations, the person should be told very bluntly that her refusal could result in death. The threat of death is sometimes necessary before such a person does what is required in these medical situations.

In a strange way, this "doubting Thomas" sometimes responds to humor or a bit of sarcasm. The latter is what she expects from others, since sincerity is simply not believed by her. It is interesting to experiment with this type of personality to see what works best. Try some ways of dealing with her, but do not waste time being excessively logical.

Example 7

Much of what is said about the paranoid personality can be said about the narcissistic person. He has no appreciation of kind and gentle ways. He is grasping and will take advantage of people. Hurting other individuals does not seem to produce guilt in him, as he has a sense of entitlement. It matters little what you have done for him thus far. He seems to have the attitude, "What have you done for me lately?" You win no points with him by being very considerate. Rather, a firm approach is best, being careful that you protect others from the narcissist to the extent that you can. Occasionally, you may have to rescue another congregant from the wiles of the narcissistic person.

The avoidant, dependent, and schizoid personalities usually do not present special problems to the clergy. They ask little and expect little, except perhaps for the overly dependent person, who sometimes may expect too much attention. But, generally these persons are not as troublesome to the clergyperson or to your congregants as the other personality types.

PERSONALITY TYPES AND THE CLERGY

It is important to recognize the different personality types and to appreciate the characteristics that make them unique. If you have some understanding and awareness of the possible variations in personality, your work with congregants will be easier.

The main problem that we all have in working with different people is that we begin dealing with each person in our usual accustomed style, which depends on our unique personality. Changing our style slightly to account for a particular personality type can make a tremendous difference in the effectiveness of our work. You cannot deal with every person the same way. Being sweet and gentle with a person with a paranoid or aggressive personality does not work well. Calming a hysterical person by speaking gently and listening helps, but you cannot deal with others in this manner and expect success.

An obsessive-compulsive personality does much better working with details. The histrionic person enjoys being in a crowd and performing. Some aggressive individuals do well raising funds for important causes, but you would not want them to deal with delicate interpersonal situations.

Tailoring the personality to the situation may take some thought, but it is a worthwhile skill to hone. In addition to following the previous advice, it is also interesting to try your skill at getting along with the various personalities that are present in any congregation. You can do this successfully by paying attention to the person and altering your involvement according to how you read him or her.

Another variation on this theme is seen in work with the elderly. Although this issue was discussed in Chapter 9, "Organic Mental Disorders," it bears repeating. When a mother or father is of the age at which they are dependent on their adult children, a conflict situation often occurs. I have counseled many families with such problems. It is often difficult for an adult to relate to his or her aged mother by seeing her as an emotionally dependent child instead of a rational mother. Often the confusion and fears of the aged are seen by adult children as real concerns that must be dealt with in concrete ways. For example, I have seen adult children try to meet each need that the parent requests, as though all requests have equal value. It is as though every parental demand must be met regardless of how impractical or irrational the demand might be. Finances must be gone over in detail, bills must be paid on a certain date, and water leaks in the house are a major tragedy. Minor concerns that were handled with dispatch at a younger age become major problems with the aged. Personality traits only dimly seen in the past now become prominent.

There are times when elderly parents must be handled as though they were children, especially when they become senile, confused, and irrational. To manage them otherwise keeps the adult children in a constantly tense and upset state of mind. Often, the children have guilt feelings when dealing with their parents this way and need counseling for this.

If variety is the spice of life, your congregation will provide lots of spice with their diverse personality styles and approaches to life. The skill with which you are able to handle the diversity of individuals in your congregation will to a large extent determine your effectiveness as a pastor. Furthermore, attending to the different personalities will provide a rich experience for you in what is, by its very nature, a difficult task. It must become a labor of love. But when you labor in the vineyards of love, it is useful to understand something about the persons with whom you are working.

Chapter 11

The Psychological Effects of Loss

Loss is everybody's business, and whether large or small, losses occur constantly. Now and then, in the practice of psychotherapy with one of my patients, things just do not work out very well, and I sense an imminent loss. The sessions seem to progress okay, but the chemistry between the patient and myself is wrong. Whatever the reason, I tell myself that a psychotherapist cannot expect to be able to help everyone–a great rationalization, with an element of truth. Meanwhile, the patient may politely say he or she would rather see someone else or is now feeling better and needs no further therapy. If done in this manner, we both save face. However, for me, there is still a sense of loss.

The loss felt in such a situation is usually mild, unless it were to occur frequently. If it did, I would seriously have to ask myself if I were working in the right field. Similarly, when a close friend is not enthusiastic about my good fortune, I may feel mildly let down. These are, indeed, mild but not unimportant instances of loss. Individuals who are not emotionally sensitive would not even notice or experience such events as loss.

I am certain that as a member of the clergy you experience similar losses. No clergyperson pleases all of his or her congregants all of the time. How could you? Each member of your congregation has a different background and a variety of personal and spiritual needs. Each person is at a particular stage of development spiritually, morally, and emotionally. My psychological and spiritual needs are different now from what they were 20 or 30 years ago. What I expect as a congregant now is quite at variance from previous years.

When you fail to meet the needs of some members in your flock, you may also notice a degree of loss. I would regard these reactions as quite normal, but I know a few clergypersons who are bothered severely by their inability to meet everyone's needs.

Compare the effects of these mild losses to what we experience with major losses. Life is full of tragedies. Accidents, serious illness, natural catastrophes, and many other events elicit a very real awareness of loss to anyone.

Are all losses the same in their effect? In some sense they are. However, objectively they may manifest themselves very differently in various people. Some persons handle major illness with dispatch. They seem to go through the stresses of illness or the death of a loved one in a way that is quite admirable. Others, in contrast, appear to be in extreme emotional pain for extended periods when loss occurs.

One of my physician friends told me some time ago that he had two patients who were diagnosed as having the same malignant cancer at about the same time. They were both facing death in one year. One patient obsessed about death and became very depressed throughout the course of his illness. In spite of reading all about his disease and researching it thoroughly, he felt no better. The other man required little attention, went about his business, and lived his life as fully as possible. The response of these men to the identical illness and the anticipated loss of life was entirely different. Both men died at about the same time, having handled the threat of dying in very individual and unique ways.

DEFENDING AGAINST LOSS

Caregivers, in whatever role they may work, have always been aware of what happens to individuals when they lose something that is of value to them. This is especially evident in the health field, where the loss of function or loss of life is encountered all too often. When major illness strikes or a patient is dying, the emotions are varied and extreme. And although physicians, nurses, clergy, and family members have always had an idea of what to expect, it had never been elucidated very well and clearly stated.

Then came the excellent book, *On Death and Dying* by Elisabeth Kübler-Ross. In it she gave a detailed version of the defenses that most persons normally experience when they are dying and are facing the ultimate loss of life itself. Much earlier, Freud wrote a significant book on a related subject; it was titled *Mourning and Melancholia*. He attempted to define the differences and similarities between these two very human experiences. He pointed out that in both mourning and in melancholia, there was a substantial repression of anger that was not expressed. That is, anger was denied. And, in working with depressed patients and those with pathological grief reactions, it is very important to recognize this factor and deal with it in psychotherapy.

Although he was a pioneer in this area, Freud did not go on to describe the other defenses that the individual experiences when confronting the possibility of death or dealing with the death of the departed. These defenses were very well elucidated by Kübler-Ross in her book. She describes five stages that the dying individual goes through at one time or another. The stages are not necessarily sequential, nor do they last an equal amount of time. Furthermore, the length of time that any person remains in a given stage varies considerably from one person to another. In general, they are as follows.

Denial

When first confronted with the threat of death, most persons will react to the shock with the defense of denial. They will say to themselves and others that it simply cannot be true (e.g., "It cannot be happening to me"). The impending death is not emotionally accepted. In contrast, there are some people who are realists and seem to deny little. They confront loss with an acceptance and equanimity that is unusual. But for most of us, denial serves a good purpose as an initial defense when we first encounter impending death.

Denial appears to be necessary for our survival. It is literally impossible to think of dying during every waking moment, even if it is imminent. The mind has a way of repressing even the most difficult situations. I have known individuals who have become ill with cancer but were never told that the disease existed, nor did the person ever ask. This happened to one of my friends. Neither his physician not his family told him that he had cancer. He had major surgery, lost considerable weight, and apparently did not become curious enough about his deteriorating condition to ask what was really wrong. His family felt that he could not bear the news that he had cancer, and so it was never discussed. But neither did he ever ask about the diagnosis.

It appears that some individuals do not want to know about their illness while others cannot deny reality to this extent and must know what is confronting them.

Anger

Upon realizing the full impact of what is happening, the dying person may become very angry. This emotion is not necessarily rational, but may be directed at innocent bystanders, be they family members or other caretakers. Sometimes the source of such anger comes from the fact that others are not suffering like the affected person who, meanwhile, is asking the question, "Why me? Why do I have to suffer like this?"

Another reason for anger is the thought of the unfulfilled life. Some ambitious folk have goals that they wish to reach during their lifetime; they become angry when anything gets in their way, especially serious illness, which often cannot be manipulated and controlled.

Anger can also emanate from the thought of leaving loved ones and from giving up meaningful relationships and pleasures long enjoyed. Some individuals never leave this stage and eventually die angry. They are not able to progress through the other stages and are not able to accept the inevitable. For most, this stage of anger is felt at the beginning and occurs intermittently throughout the duration of the illness although it usually diminishes with time.

Depression

As Freud pointed out, anger can be converted to depression when it is turned inward upon the self. As long as the anger in the first stage is directed outward toward others, toward fate, God, or anywhere else, depression will not occur. But when this mental operation fails, depression usually follows. It may appear that the person has simply given up and is doing a "slow burn" (withholding anger).

Depression can be of variable intensity, from mild to severe, and may include suicidal ideation or actual attempts at suicide. Someone with a severe illness may regard the news of impending death as the last straw in his mental burden. He may view this as the time to hasten his exit from life, rather than endure the anticipated pain and suffering. This phenomenon is occurring with increasing frequency among the elderly, when the increased signs of aging appear with or without significant serious illness. In recent years, as the population is living longer, the suicide rate among the elderly has increased remarkably.

Whether it occurs in short intervals or becomes chronic, depression, with its inevitable feelings of hopelessness, may take a considerable toll on the individual as well as the family, who may try in vain to raise the spirits of the depressed person. It is at this stage that the clergy should appreciate the value of simply *listening* to the depressed individual. The benefits of simply listening, with little or no comment, cannot be overestimated. Depressive thinking is repetitive and predictable–the mood low and hopeless. Although it is difficult to listen to a depressed person for long periods of time, a sympathetic listener often can be a great comfort and support for the sufferer during this most difficult period.

Needless to say, if the depressed individual expresses suicidal ideas, he should be evaluated by a psychiatrist in order to determine the need for medication to help him through this stage.

The clergy as well as the family should also be aware of the fact that a certain amount of firmness in dealing with depression is also in order. Firmness on the part of the caregiver reassures the depressed person that he is cared for; it can help mobilize his other defenses to energize him and hasten his recovery. For example, I have often seen family members become impatient with the inability of the depressed individual to help himself. Caregivers have feelings too; they become annoyed or overtly angry at the lack of response to their suggestions. When this happens, I advise the family to be firm. It helps to fix their anger on a specific target and also has a way of stimulating the depressed person.

"Don't let him lie in bed until noon. Get him up the same time every morning. Get him to move his muscles. The worst thing for him to do is lie awake in bed contemplating his fate." Suggestions like these are of help, and I use them regularly with the depressed person's family.

Listening attentively and being firm are the two most useful tools the caregiver can employ in dealing with depression in a family member who has recently been told of an impending loss.

Bargaining

When a person is depressed, she is in no mood for bargaining. She is silently angry, feeling too hopeless, and she sees no way out of her situation. At some point, it occurs to her, that if she strikes a bargain with God or fate or life itself, perhaps she can emerge victorious. She says, "God, if you save me from this disease, I will devote my life to a good cause"—or a similar bargain. It is a quid pro quo with God, or whomever, to work out a miracle in return for some good deed. Bargaining must occur in the climate of possibilities. When the agreement is reached in the mind of the bargainer, a certain degree of equanimity results. From here, the person can proceed to the final stage of resolution.

Resolution

In some dying persons, bargaining and resolution never occur. They may remain stuck in anger or depression, unable to go forward emotionally to the next stage. But, for those who are able, the stage of resolution or acceptance is a more satisfactory level to attain. Here, the individual may say, "I no longer deny the reality of my illness and impending death. Let's see what I have to do to arrange my affairs and go about this with some pride and dignity. I accept the fact of death that comes to all of us. I wish it were not at this time, but I must accept it and deal with it."

Of course, arriving at such a mature conclusion is not without moments of regression to stages of anger and depression. No one can be so emotionally secure as to never revert to former levels of despair. But many individuals can, for the most part, attain the stage of resolution on a day-to-day basis.

It should be understood that these stages are not progressive in terms of time. As with growth and development of the child, there are stages that can be recognized, but they are not always exactly sequential. They may all occur on a given day, only to change the next day. When talking to a dying individual, it is helpful to be aware of the stage that he or she is in. It facilitates greater understanding of the person and enables you to be a better caregiver and clergyperson with your congregant.

RECOGNIZING STAGES OF GRIEF IN THE FAMILY

The stages discussed refer to the dying person. These stages are also experienced by the family and friends of the dying or deceased. It can be very useful to try to identify in these mourners the stages that are possible. In some of the survivors, there may be some or none of the stages noted. In others, all the stages may be easily seen. It depends on the emotional state of the griever, as well as the relationship to the deceased. If the loss is deeply felt, the stages are likely to occur. If the loss is mild or perchance welcomed, the stages may not be present. At times, the griever is so distraught that he may remain in one stage for a prolonged time. This happened to one of my patients.

A couple came to me for marital counseling. They had battled for 30 years about their children, the lack of mutual satisfaction in the marriage, and many other problems. I tried to help them, and we were experiencing some success. In spite of the anger and hostility displayed in the course of marriage, these partners had a basic love for each other and at intervals really enjoyed their relationship.

It was not long after counseling was ended, that Mary, the wife, suddenly died in an accident. The husband, Joe, was very distraught, deeply depressed, and seemed unable to come out of it. He could not work and was not able to enjoy anything; his thoughts turned to hopelessness and despair. After six months of depression, he was no better; in fact, he was suicidal. He returned to my office, this time for psychotherapy and medication to combat his depression.

Joe expressed his deep love for his wife. He minimized the marital stress that had existed and put Mary on a pedestal in an unreal fashion. In his eyes, she was now ready for sainthood; she was just about the most wonderful person that had ever existed. He could not utter a negative word about her. The man was obviously denying his anger toward his deceased wife, and the result was sustained depression. Such denial is not an uncommon dynamic in the survivors of a loved one. It represents a failure to remember the departed as a human being with assets as well as human failings. It is also a failure to come to terms with the anger toward that loved one for suddenly leaving, for interrupting the relationship, and for putting all of the family responsibilities on the remaining partner. In most of us, this anger is real and normal when death occurs, and it must be recognized and given some ventilation.

After weeks of psychotherapy and medication, Joe felt a bit better able to cope. He was no longer suicidal and was able to return to work. I had to remind him of the fights, to which I was witness, when he and Mary had come to me for marital counseling. Gradually, he admitted to feelings of anger toward her and was able to see Mary in a more realistic light—a good, caring, faithful person, but with human faults like all of us.

In some marriages the denial of anger is immense, and the person remaining may have a chronic depression that never resolves. Such a clinical picture is seen most often in the elderly, usually after a long marriage, but it can also occur in younger persons if the emotional factors involving death are not satisfactorily played out. It constantly amazes me how differently people handle death and dying—certainly the most difficult of losses that humans have to endure.

Lesser Losses

These defenses, which are clearly defined by Kübler-Ross, are seen in the dying person as he or she approaches the ultimate loss—of life itself—when the very essence or ground of being is threatened.

But what of lesser losses? These we can experience frequently. Loss of control of our emotions and loss of power, wealth, or self-esteem are familiar to us all at one time or another. As I am writing, many young people are suffering the loss of or separation from a loved one in the war in the Middle East. And as we experience these or other losses, we go through similar defense mechanisms in order to cope with the loss.

At times, the mind runs through the defenses rapidly or sporadically. At other times, some defenses are skipped. Every time we experience a loss, we do not necessarily deny it or get deeply depressed. We may simply become angry, grouse about it for a while, or even obsess about it, but we do not go through other stages. Bargaining may not occur in response to our lesser losses and usually occurs only in severe types of loss. Instead, we often use the defense of rationalization to heal our losses.

With rationalization we allow that some things occur as part of living. Losses are accepted as unavoidable or to be expected. Through rationalization we justify our losses; we make them bearable rather than feel the anger or depression associated with loss. In rationalization, we give socially acceptable reasons for our losses and thus minimize their effects.

Examples of Loss

Loss at Work

Anne was an executive secretary at her firm, had worked hard for many years, and had a successful career. She had never suffered a loss at work. Anne was getting close to retirement; she had received a raise in pay each year. But this time, as the end of the year approached, she heard nothing of an increase in pay. She inquired about her financial status and was told that no pay increase would be forthcoming for that year. The company was not in bad shape, nor was she given cogent reasons for the failure to receive a raise. In addition, there were no financial concerns in her life; she had adequate resources and could have easily retired on the spot and lived comfortably.

But this news hit her as a severe loss. Anne was not able to sleep through the night, lost 15 pounds, became physically ill, was very depressed, and could not concentrate. At one point, she had to stop working because of her symptoms.

It took some months to treat Anne's depression. She remained at home for several weeks while I counseled her in my office and gave her antidepressants. Gradually, she accepted her loss, put it in perspective, and was able to rise above it and feel normal again.

I have seen similar reactions in individuals who failed to receive a promotion. It is often experienced as a loss in position or prestige. Anger and depression follow, sometimes requiring psychotherapeutic treatment.

Early Retirement

In recent years, a common cause of deeply felt loss is the area of early retirement, a relatively new phenomenon. One day, a man named Jack came to see me because of a deep depression that he could not shake. Jack had been employed with the same company for a number of years. He enjoyed his work as a salesman, but he enjoyed the camaraderie with his fellow workers even more. To Jack, going to work was a tonic. Although he was able to relax on vacations, he never minded returning to his job because it was so much a part of him. He never thought of retirement; it seemed years away, even though he was 60 years old. Besides, he had so many interests and friends that retirement would be no problem.

Then, suddenly, without any forewarning, he was retired prematurely. He could not believe it (denial). He became alternately angry at his superiors and depressed by the tremendous loss that he felt. No longer would he be able to have lunch with the boys, savor the latest jokes, and enjoy the mutual kidding and card playing on the train in the morning. He could not bear to think of it. He had been the life of the party at the office; now he literally had no audience. He did not simply lose his job; he lost the "whole package." Even though he had a devoted wife and fine children, his work had been his life. He was so identified with his job that without it he felt useless.

When this kind of loss occurs, a person is without purpose. Some may say, "It feels like the bottom has fallen out." Jack had suffered previous losses before, but this was by far the worst. The anger centered around the feeling of betrayal. After all, Jack had been a loyal worker. He had performed well. But the company was retrenching in the way that companies do; it was not a personal thing as far as his boss was concerned. Jack, however, took it very personally and even became a bit paranoid about it. Mostly, he was depressed. And, as often happens in these circumstances, he started to have ideas of suicide. Life just did not seem worth it. He had counted on many more years of work, a larger pension, and more time to accumulate enough money on which to retire. He felt that all was lost; he exaggerated his financial situation while his wife tried to reassure him that they had adequate funds to get along nicely.

Jack was not an easy patient. He required hospitalization to protect him from suicide. Antidepressants did not help as much as they do usually do. Finally, Jack had to be transferred to another physician, who gave him electroconvulsive shock therapy (ECT).

Following the ECT, Jack needed counseling to help him with plans for a new life–a life apart from his lost job. He had to find a new place to enjoy friends, feel needed, and be involved.

Loss Experienced with Divorce

Divorce is a common reason for the feelings of loss. Even when the two parties are both resigned to divorce and welcome it, there are still times when the divorced person reflects, in a moment of nostalgia, on some of the good times when things were going along well. There are the days remembered when the children were young, when hopes and aspirations were fresh, when nothing seemed impossible. Then the reality of a failed marriage sets in, with its guilt, ambivalence, and heartache. And there are always the children caught in the middle, between parents who are uncertain of their way, torn in their loyalties, and still trying to be all that they hoped to be as parents.

I have seen divorced couples who could not stand to be divorced. They began dating each other soon after the divorce occurred and tried to rebuild the relationship. Most often this attempt is doomed to failure. If a couple had not been able to work out their feelings about each other in the years before, there is usually little chance that it can be done after the trauma of a divorce, with its mutual maligning and castigation, which is urged on by aggressive attorneys. Of course, there are instances when miracles happen even in the matrimonial area, but they are rare. In the arena of love, hope certainly springs eternal. People do not like to fail, whether at marriage or in any other of life's ventures.

Loss of Power

When one ascends to power, it is an exhilarating experience. I witnessed it firsthand when my wife, who after two attempts was successfully elected to the U.S. Congress. On the very first day that she walked into her office, she was greeted by a ringing phone. It was so early that the staff had as yet not arrived. A constituent was calling about an international incident that involved a family member. In order to deal with this problem, the new congresswoman had to call the State Department and sequentially reach higher levels of command. Toward evening she was on the phone with the Secretary of State. In their conversation, he recommended that she call the family in regard to the matter and tell them what was known of the situation. She politely told the Secretary that the call would mean much more to the family if he did the calling; he agreed to make the call.

When I heard this story, the power aspects impressed me; one day my wife was a housewife/teacher/mother, and the next day she was making suggestions to the Secretary of State as to how to proceed in his role. Wow! What sudden elevation to power!

By contrast, in the last ten years, I have seen the mighty fall, popular members of congress and senators defeated, governors done in by the voters. We can all recall Watergate and the political demise of Richard Nixon. To fall from power is a psychologically difficult loss. Some handle it with considerable rationalization and denial. Others are not so fortunate. Some people who lose power need to be treated for depression or other emotional illnesses although in the political arena, we are not always privy to this information.

Whether the loss of power is in the realm of status, influence, or role, it feels the same when the loss occurs. The ego really takes a hit. Some egos are resilient; others are not. Some persons have a wonderful group of supportive people around them, and others have to stand alone.

One mental mechanism that seems to help many people with loss is the defense of projection. Here the politician blames the voters, the unemployed blame the company, the rejected lover blames the one who rejected him or her, and the child blames the parent. It is a way of unconsciously finding fault in the other person, a fault that has its origin in the self. It absolves one of responsibility for what has happened. And, in spite of the fact that the pathology begins in the self, it psychologically helps the person to survive the event of loss.

Loss Through Separation

Our first significant loss of major security occurs upon entering nursery school or kindergarten. We are a long way from home during the first day at school. Some children cry when their parent leaves; others are in a state of panic. Still others acclimate themselves to the new situation very well. But, the first day of school is the big separation from home–the ultimate source of security for most children.

When I was a psychiatric consultant to public schools, I frequently saw children with "school phobia." The name implies that the child is afraid of school. Actually, more often than not, the child is not afraid of school but is fearful of leaving home. A separation anxiety occurs with symptoms of nausea, vomiting, malaise, and general anxiety complaints. When a doctor is consulted, no organic disease is found. Often, the parents do not initially accept this finding and go to other doctors in an attempt to uncover some pathology. At times, the illness is so severe that teenage children do not attend school for months at a time. I have examined more than one adolescent who, because of a school phobia, was not able to attend classes for all of high school.

The same phenomenon occurs with the homesickness of children who attend summer camp or even the first attempt at going to college. Those afflicted with separation anxiety suffer severe panic, which disappears entirely upon returning home. Adults who have agoraphobia (severe panic when in unfamiliar places or inability to escape from certain situations) often have a history of separation anxiety in childhood. The attachment to home for some persons cannot be underestimated. The security of the familiar, of being surrounded by family and friends and by inanimate objects that provide support, is of enormous importance. To some individuals, it is absolutely crucial; to others, it has no great hold.

I have met those who speak lovingly of their possessions, as though they were dear friends. We usually are not so aware of the importance of our home environment until we are away from it for a time. On the other hand, there are those who welcome change, who are restless about staying in one place, or who are born wanderers. Their comfortable environment seems to travel with them. They make easy adjustments that others would find difficult. Some of us need many familiar props for support. Others need few and get along very well on little that is familiar. I think I was such a person in my youth, but as I grow older, the familiar and the creature comforts have become more important to me, and I am less adventurous.

Many times I have had patients tell me that the depression that they were experiencing began when they moved from one house to another. Sometimes, the depression had started even before the move in anticipation of the change and the loss of the familiar.

Some individuals react adversely to changes of environment such as being hospitalized. This is most obvious in the elderly, who may be bordering on organic mental disease. While still at home, an elderly person may be mentally intact. Upon being hospitalized for a physical reason, the patient may suddenly become grossly psychotic with disorientation, recent memory loss, and even hallucinations. I have witnessed this on a number of occasions. Such symptoms generally clear up rapidly, particularly if the patient can be sent home quickly. Here, the sudden loss of the familiar environment plus the stress of being hospitalized can be enough to cause a drastic change in mental performance.

While in the military service, I saw many young men who had a variety of neurotic symptoms that resulted from being unable to endure the stress of military life. Most of all, they were bothered by the absence of the familiar props of home, friends, and family, even if their relationship with family and friends was not optimal.

Loss of Function

Perhaps the most obvious loss of our ability to function is when accidents occur. Part of the reason is the sudden onset. One day one is healthy and performing well and the next day one is in bed, totally dependent upon caregivers. Such an event is especially difficult for the person who prides herself in her independence and ability to go it alone. For example, when the aggressive, type-A personality gets immobilized in bed with a compound fracture, she becomes very difficult to manage. The person is demanding, angry, impatient, and intolerant of everyone. The type-A personality generally remains angry throughout the confinement, although some depression may also be present. Only at the end of the period of immobility is there any lessening of the anger toward the loss.

A more common reaction to loss of function is depression. It may be mixed with anger. Some bargaining may occur before a resolution is finally reached. However, in some persons, the depression and anger remain for long periods of time. In the case of accidents, this is complicated in our society by the fact that the victims of accidents are frequently awarded large sums of money by insurance companies via courts of law. There is a financial incentive to stay ill and appear to be more incapacitated than necessary. It is amazing, in some cases, what miraculous recoveries occur after the insurance company settles with the patient. The power and importance of money in our litigious society can never be overestimated.

Aside from any financial motivation to remain ill, many people do not suffer loss well. This occurs especially with individuals who have always prided themselves in their self-sufficiency. To be able to perform physically in many areas is very gratifying to the ego, particularly in those who have placed a high priority on this ability. It is difficult for such a person to sit and think about past accomplishments while mourning present deficiencies. In addition, the inability of the patient to perform in the same old way may cause severe difficulties in relationships with family members. I have seen such situations lead to severe marital dysfunction and divorce. It is not easy to live with someone who continues to mourn the loss of previous abilities. On the other hand, family members may not be able to adjust well to the absence of services that the injured member had performed. The anger on the part of the family may further the depression of the patient since he or she now has both the loss due to the injury in addition to the lack of support of the family.

I recently experienced a loss firsthand. Several months ago, I had the dubious pleasure of needing cardiac surgery. A defective heart valve, which I have had since birth, became calcified and had to be replaced. It was the first time that I ever experienced any kind of hospitalization or surgery. It was not an experience that I shall cherish although the care was excellent, and I could not have asked for more qualified and competent caregivers.

In my medical readings about depression, I had noted that in the old days of cardiac surgery, about 30 percent of patients experienced depression postoperatively. With increased experience, the surgery teams have been able to reduce the number to about 5 percent. I did not intend to be included in this number, and, indeed, my spirits were good in the weeks following surgery. Having been always fond of exercise and physical fitness, I did not consider it an imposition to be asked to exercise regularly. All went well for about the first three months. Then, one day, I attempted to ski at a familiar ski area–down the same trails that I used to "shush" without stopping. It took me five times as long to get down the slopes because I had to stop to catch my breath. I did not find this an exhilarating and ego-enhancing experience. Furthermore, in my regular exercise routine, I had reached a plateau and found that I was having difficulty attaining new levels. It was at this time that a mild depression set in, which was not enough to interfere with work, but I knew it was there. I had become aware of the loss of physical abilities that had been precious to me.

Fortunately, this period was short-lived; I have reached new ground, and I am gradually gaining more strength. My spirits are renewed, even if I never get to the level that I had been at before the surgery. One has to accept some compromises in life.

DEALING WITH LOSS

How does one cope with loss? It depends on the loss and the degree to which the loss is felt. A loss to one person may not be a loss to another. It is our interpretation of the significance of the loss that is important. To some, even small losses have the potential for causing severe symptoms such as depression. Furthermore, one loss following upon another and another may be the reason for the person being unable to withstand the pressure.

If the loss is felt as mild, there are a number of avenues to take. It helps to ventilate the loss to sympathetic friends. Just getting the pain out in the open may be all that is necessary. For most people, a loss hurts more if the knowledge of the loss is withheld. We are social beings with a need to express our pain.

While doing so, our natural defenses are likely to kick in, thereby rescuing us from the effects of loss. We rationalize, as I did in my experiences after cardiac surgery. We repress (unconsciously forget) about our losses or get angry at someone for causing the loss and thus project the blame onto someone or something. One way or another, our defenses may help us handle the loss appropriately without causing us further pain.

It may be useful to ask certain questions regarding a specific loss. Have you considered making changes in your life that could affect how a loss impinges on you? What advantages would accrue from changes made? What can you do about the situation that you are not doing? Attempting to answer such questions can help one find ways to overcome a psychological loss.

Ultimately, I must take responsibility for the losses that occur to me. Although others may assist and make life easier for me, it is my ability to adjust to the losses in life that will make the difference regarding how I feel. The dependent person expects others to make up for what she is not able to do or does not want to do.

If the loss to an individual is moderate, she is likely to go through the various stages that Kübler-Ross has suggested. Denial may not be a large part of the process, but anger and depression will be present in varying degrees. If these two residuals of loss are temporary, there is no need for further concern. However, if weeks and months go by and anger and depression persist without resolution, psychotherapy and perhaps medication become necessary.

In some cases, the loss produces severe reactions. A good example is grieving the loss of a loved one. It is common to see the survivor react excessively but for a short time. I have heard of more than one grieving spouse who was uncontrollable at the funeral of his spouse, and everyone witnessed his pain. When he remarried six months later, his friends were confounded at his quick recovery. Usually, recovery from loss takes longer. Most of us experiencing loss react more moderately but for a longer time.

In *The Grief Recovery Handbook* by John W. James and Frank Cherry, the authors describe one type of griever as having "admirable restraint and poise" and refer to such reactions as "Academy Award" recoveries. These individuals may later have prolonged states of regression that may last years and can include clinical depression.

Still others, regardless of the type of loss, react with severe symptoms. More often than not, the person who does not handle loss well ends up with a severe depression. I have had patients react in this way regardless of the kind of loss—business failure, early retirement, loss of a loved one, or other reasons. If the depression is deep enough, the person may become suicidal. Obviously, in such severe conditions, professional assistance is required. The use of antidepressants can often make a considerable difference in shortening the recovery period and preventing suicide. Hospitalization and the use of electroconvulsive shock therapy may be necessary if medication is ineffective. In this regard, the question is sometimes asked, "How can physical treatments like medication or ECT help a psychological state such as grieving?" The answer lies in the fact that in severe states of depression, there are physical changes in the nervous system. The normal neurotransmitters in the brain are depleted, resulting in the clinical syndrome of depression. When this is treated, the neurotransmitters are restored with subsequent clinical improvement. For further information on this subject see Chapter 3, "Biochemistry, Mental Illness, and Medication."

For the person who is grieving the loss of a loved one, I would recommend the previously mentioned book *The Grief Recovery Handbook*. Among other things, the authors assert that we are taught to acquire things in life and are not taught to lose them, regardless of whether these are inanimate objects or significant others. They also write about common myths in our culture that concern grieving:

• We must replace what was lost with something or somebody.
• It is best to grieve alone.
• It is best to bury feelings.
• Time will cure you.
• One should regret the past and wish it were different.
• Because of past losses, it does not pay to trust.

The authors present a specific plan for dealing with grief. They suggest that the griever should not try to grieve alone. Rather, he or she should deal with grief in association with someone else who is also engaged in mourning.

LOSS AND THE CLERGY

The subject of loss and grieving is familiar territory to the clergy. My guess is that the clergy deal with grieving more than any other profession (including physicians) except, of course, for undertakers. Even the latter group is taking more responsibility for mourners by giving them information about grieving and organizing groups to deal with loss.

Although most members of the clergy are familiar with the literature on death and dying spearheaded by Kübler-Ross, clergypersons may not be as aware of how even minor losses can cause great distress in congregants. For example, the death of a pet to me might be a minor loss in the scheme of things, but to an ardent pet lover it might represent a much greater loss. This is especially true when the pet owner symbolically embraces the animal with the affection usually reserved for a child.

A person between the ages of 50 and 60 generally accepts the fact that he has lived most of his life, and that he will not progress much beyond the present situation professionally, socially, or financially. But others, sensing a loss of power, energy, position, or prestige, may feel a loss that overwhelms them. The popular midlife crisis contains many elements, among which is the sense that life is slipping away before one has tasted enough of it. Drug abuse, gambling, extramarital affairs, or job changes are variously used to cope with the impending sense of loss. Such acting-out behavior, although temporarily soothing to the stressed individual, does not solve basic issues in the long-term.

What can the clergy do with the congregant who is suffering loss? Unless the loss is obvious, the person will not say that she is dealing with loss. The complaint may occur in a disguised fashion. One has to look for the loss when a married congregant announces that she has fallen in love with someone else. The underlying loss may be far more important than the newfound gain. To review what may be obvious to many experienced clergypersons, I would suggest the following:

1. Listen carefully to your congregant. His or her loss may be hidden behind a smoke screen that may include physical complaints.

2. Allow sufficient ventilation. The real issues seldom are expressed in the first few minutes. Time is very important in your counseling role. If you do not have enough time on a given day, arrange counseling for another hour when you are not rushed. The emotional support of a sympathetic listener cannot be overestimated. Healing can often occur without many words being spoken.

3. Ask questions rather than give immediate answers. Explore and attempt to clarify the problem; do not give quick suggestions.

4. Use others in your congregation to help support those in need. If you know of groups attending to the needs of those who are mourning, refer your congregant to the appropriate place.

5. If your congregant is distressed beyond your ability or comfort to help, refer to a professional who can deal with the situation. This, of course, is a judgment call. I have met clergypersons with rescue fantasies who never referred congregants to anyone. They preferred to do it all alone as if no one else could possibly understand. Such arrogance and misdirected faith did more harm than good to the involved congregants. It helps to know your limits and recognize when you are working beyond your limits in the counseling area.

It is my opinion that religious faith and the supportive help of the clergy do much to hold together our society, even in an age when there is much religion bashing and denial of the need for a religious experience. The clergy deal with matters of life and death on a daily basis and are always present to deal with our serious losses. It is easy for the public to underestimate the valuable work that each member of the clergy is doing for his or her people. Unfortunately, our society gives few plaudits to the hard work that the clergy does in maintaining the moral fabric of our culture.

Chapter 12

Sexual Problems in Our Culture

Since the days of Adam and Eve, humans have been delighted, ecstatic, tormented, and perplexed by their sexual urges. King David had to have yet one more sexual conquest even if it meant arranging to have Bathsheba's husband killed in battle. From the sirens of Greek mythology to the beauty queens of Hollywood, the mystery of sexuality has been a subject of endless interest and fascination.

In humans and in animals, the sexual urge is persistent, at times even obsessive. Is it any surprise that caution is often thrown to the wind and humans blithely overlook sexually transmitted diseases and even the threat of death in order to satisfy sexual desires? And consider how sex is used, not just for the relief of sexual tension and the pleasure that it affords, but for power, for meeting sadistic and masochistic needs, for elevating self-esteem, for satisfying dependent and aggressive needs, and for obtaining control and power over others.

I have occasionally made the remark to my patients, "God really knew what he was doing when he created the sexual urge. He made sexuality an overwhelming preoccupation, an urge so strong that it virtually guaranteed that mankind would not be easily dissuaded from propagating the race."

But, there is an inherent problem in the sexual drive. Frequently, it consists of a driving lust, a blind pursuit of a sexual object, often with little regard for consequences or circumstances. At other times, individuals have the ability to analyze their actions, to assess the appropriateness of their sexual intentions, and to decide whether their goals are culturally and psychologically acceptable. Furthermore, humans have the need for intimacy, the need to feel closely

related to one or more persons, for friends and family, and especially the need to have one person with whom to relate in the most
confidential, personal, and intimate way. The problem, then, consists in harmonizing or integrating the lustful, cognitive, and intimacy needs that each person possesses.

Some persons are capable of intimacy with others but fail to have
feelings of lust. Others are very aware of their lustful urges, but
ignore or are unable to express intimacy needs. This dichotomy is
most evident in early adolescence when the blossoming teenager
recognizes the "good (idealized) girls and the bad girls," or "good
(idealized) boys and the bad boys." Sexuality is usually associated
first with the bad, rather than the idealized images of each gender.
This conflict is eloquently portrayed in *The Odyssey* in which the
sirens call the sailors to sexuality, while the faithful Penelope pines
at home for her idealized love.

In mythology as in organized religion, the dichotomy between
lust and intimacy has been highlighted. The idealized image of man
or woman offered by organized religions is often in stark contrast to
the seamy side of sex that is portrayed in literature and in the
theater. Many individuals grow to adulthood still preoccupied with
this problem, having never resolved the lust versus intimacy issue.
In marriage this can be a difficult problem. For example, I have
seen men or women who have intimate emotional relationships with
their marriage partners. "He's my best friend, but I cannot think of
him sexually." "She's a wonderful person in every way, but sexual
feelings just don't exist." An example of this is the couple that I
interviewed at a mental health clinic. They were very much in love,
enjoyed each other's company, were very supportive of each other,
and liked the same activities. In 20 years they had never consum-
mated the marriage: not a single successful sexual encounter had
occurred in all that time. Other than a few attempts initially, there
had been no sexual contact for all those years. The husband had a
primary impotence that appeared incurable. His wife had sexual
feelings at times, but she said that after so many years of no sexual
activity, she had lost interest in sex. But she felt that her emotional
needs were being met, and she elected to remain married. Although
this is an extreme example of the failure to fuse intimacy and lust,

such cases do exist. (For further reading on this subject, see works by Harry Stack Sullivan.)

There is another problem related to lust and intimacy—the problem of varying sexual and emotional needs. It is a common observation that the sexual urges of men are more compulsive than those of women. Evidence for this can be found statistically in the research of Kinsey. It is also evident in the paraphilias, the sexual abnormalities that will be discussed later. If one were to look at the incidence of paraphilia in the general population, it would be evident that such abnormalities as exhibitionism, fetishism, and sadism are notably more common in males than in females, in which they rarely occur. There is a strong element of compulsion in all such abnormal sexual behavior.

Furthermore, in the psychological nature of women in our culture, the homebuilding, childrearing, and security needs appear to be greater. This may well be true in virtually all cultures if these needs are more biologically driven. Of course, it can be argued that the different needs in women and men are culturally determined. But regardless of how it comes about, these factors are at work in our everyday lives. It is not uncommon for a man to enter marriage with the expectation that his compulsive need for sexual gratification be met, only to find out that his spouse is much more interested in fulfilling her homebuilding or security needs. In contrast, I have met more than a few female patients who were very distressed by their husband's preoccupation with vocational pursuits and their own simultaneous lack of interest in the sexual aspects of marriage. And so it goes. These are not easy issues to resolve.

RECENT CHANGES

Since the 1960s and 1970s, there has been a noticeable increase in sexual freedom, which has eliminated some problems and increased others. While increased sexual freedom allowed for less inhibition in the expression of sexuality, it is my observation that many individuals have become more confused by complications in their lives as a result of multiple sexual encounters. In spite of increased sexual freedom, there appears to be little or no increase in level of satisfaction or contentment. Nor is there a decrease in neurotic or psychosomatic symptoms in the general population. Rather, for whatever reasons, many of these illnesses appear to have increased, contrary to what Freud might have expected. Many years ago, he speculated that the repression of sexual and aggressive impulses led to neuroses. Presumably, if these impulses were allowed freer expression, the incidence of neuroses would decline.

Furthermore, as women have become less dependent and more assertive, some men have reacted with sexual impotence (Kaplan, 1974, p. 262). As in the world of physics, when one change is made in the human equation, it has reverberating effects in the field surrounding the source of change. Also, as many men have become more overt and demanding about their sexual needs, women have been turned off by the lack of emotional considerations surrounding the sexual encounter. Instead of *solving* past sexual problems, the change in sexual mores in our culture appear to have merely *altered* the problems.

Only a few generations ago, cohabitation between unmarried persons was frowned on by society. We spoke of common law marriages that occurred mostly among the poor and uneducated. Today, sexual intimacy is more and more common in adolescence. Promiscuity and sequential sexual partnerships appear more prevalent. Living together among the young has become very common, much to the distress of many parents. To me, such arrangements are like "playing house." It has little relationship to the reality of marriage. The young persons with whom I have spoken confirm this. In fact, they have made me aware of the differences between cohabitation and the institution of marriage. The latter includes shared responsibilities of finance, property, children, the extended family, and many other commitments; it is a whole package. In marriage, the couple is in it together for better or for worse. In cohabitation, when the first problem comes along, one party or the other can simply pack his or her belongings and move on to another relationship.

The institution of marriage is so structured that it is much more binding than a simple understanding. It encourages the long haul–of solving life's problems together. And there is a payoff. The mature love, support, comfort, and pleasures of a good marriage and a close family are rewards that cannot be achieved in any other way.

THE SEXUAL DISORDERS

Sexual pathology is classified into three areas:

1. Gender identity
2. Paraphilias
3. Sexual dysfunction

The following is a general description of these disorders in sexuality, along with clinical comments about their manifestations in psychiatric practice.

Gender identity includes two aspects: psychological and biological. The former consists of a recognition of being male or female and an acceptance or at least resignation to the fact. The latter concerns sexual identity; that is, awareness of the physical external sexual characteristics, be it male or female.

One day, I saw a 14-year-old girl in my office. She told me in definitive terms that she had always thought of herself as a boy. She did everything she could to look like a boy. She always wore male clothing and a very constricting bra to hide her developing breasts. Her clear intention was to do what was necessary to have a sex change as soon as she became of age. As far as she was concerned, her sexual identity was male even though her physical characteristics were unquestionably female.

Sexual identity disturbances are affected by at least three factors:

1. Genetic influences begin in the developing fetus as early as the sixth week of pregnancy.
2. Gender identity is influenced by such things as physique, size, shape, and other physical characteristics.
3. Interaction of the child with parents, teachers, peers, and cultural factors all play a significant role in gender identity.

As a consequence of these factors, the developing person assumes a gender role in society through the various influences that affect him or her. Gender conflicts can result from parents consciously or unconsciously wishing for a child of the opposite sex. This can be observed in a home in which a parent dresses a girl in male clothing or encourages female activities for his or her male child. But such influences alone, while producing conflicts, do not cause abnormal gender identity. The exact manner in which gender disturbances evolve is still a mystery and requires much more research to understand. When manifested in adulthood or even in adolescence, a disorder of sexual identity is extremely difficult to change. Actually, in most instances there is no desire for the involved person to change the sexual identity. Feelings of being male or female are so strong that the person sees no reason to remain his or her biological sex and will often ask for a sex change operation.

THE PARAPHILIAS

The word paraphilia originates from the Greek words *para* (to go along with) and *philia* (love). A paraphilia is an extreme sexual desire involving sexual fantasies and practices that are not common in the general population. The desires and acts are compulsive in nature, and although pleasurable for the moment, usually cause considerable emotional discomfort to the paraphiliac individual. Paraphilias were formerly called perversions.

Generally, these disorders fall into three categories. In the first, the paraphiliac has an extreme sexual attraction to children or other persons who do not consent to the sexual act. In the second category, the person has an unusual attraction to objects that are related to the opposite sex. In the third, the individual has a strong desire to inflict pain or discomfort on the self or others.

The fantasies involved in the paraphilias are very persistent and chronic. They are usually associated with acting out the fantasy as well as achieving sexual excitement and orgasm. An occasional fantasy that is paraphiliac in nature would not be regarded as a disorder.

Some paraphiliacs suffer severe guilt and anxiety about their sexual preoccupations while others do not seem to be particularly upset about them. The latter type rarely consults a physician, whereas the former may come for consultation because of anxiety and fear of being discovered. Most often, the paraphiliac comes to therapy on a referral from a lawyer or from a court of law. In such instances, their anxiety is caused by a fear of arrest and incarceration. I have seen a few patients in my office who were in no legal difficulties and who genuinely wanted to make changes in their sexual proclivities. Such alterations in sexual acting out are possible, especially if the paraphilia is of late onset. For example, if a man had one or two experiences of touching his daughter in a sexually inappropriate way, he could be treated successively in psychotherapy, providing he felt motivated to do so. Likewise, exhibitionism is treatable with psychotherapy.

Paraphilia appears to be almost exclusively a male disease. Very few cases have been reported in women. But in a recent book written by Louise J. Kaplan, *The Temptations of Emma Bovary*, the author suggests that women express their disturbed sexuality in other ways, such as in eating disorders, dressing provocatively, and by shoplifting. This is an interesting idea. I think it is most evident in the problem of anorexia, where there is an attempt at hiding sexuality and denying its existence, while exhibiting the self in an unusual way—emaciated and thin. Most individuals who become paraphiliac are aware of their sexual tendencies at an early age.

Types of Paraphilias

Pedophilia

Pedophilia is an intense desire to relate to children in an overtly sexual manner. By definition, the child is young, has not attained adolescence, and is at least ten years younger than the other party involved. Those who suffer from this disorder are usually insecure, have low self-esteem, and do not have satisfactory adult sexual relations. Usually the person feels that he or she can manipulate a child toward a sexual encounter easier than another adult. Many pedophiles have a history of having been sexually molested in childhood.

In recent years, the sexual molestation of children has reached proportions not dreamed of in the past. Some of the reports are no doubt true. But, the reporting is not scientific and is actually difficult to document. In a newly published book on this subject by Dr. Richard Gardner, a well-known child psychiatrist at Columbia University, the author talks about the hysteria regarding this subject. His thesis is that the reporting of sexual molestation of children by family members is mostly true, but he doubts the statistics about pedophilia from nursery schools and day care centers. Dr. Gardner speaks from a wide experience in private practice, family therapy, and legal work. He views the present search for the pedophilic villains as similar to the Salem witch trials.

Pedophilic behavior on the part of adults usually wreaks havoc on the young and unsuspecting. It has damaged many a young person at a time when the developing ego needs all the support it can get. On the other hand, I have been surprised at the number of adult patients who have told me that they were molested as children. When asked about any permanent damage that might have accrued from such earlier experiences, they often have been unable to give any certain evidence of harm having occurred. These adults were consulting me for reasons other than sexual problems, and they had mentioned the molestation only parenthetically.

It appears that the trauma from these experiences comes via the malevolent intentions of the pedophilic in conjunction with the vulnerability of the child. The child who is least secure and most vulnerable will be the one most damaged. The more threatening the pedophilic individual is in a verbal or physical manner, the worse the effect on the child.

Why do some adults have a sexual attraction to children? One explanation has to do with the issue of control. A child is easily manipulated, easily plied with candy or toys, and easily threatened. Adult pedophiles have difficulty with self-esteem and interpersonal relationships. For them, it is much easier and less threatening to engage a child in a sexual act than to be involved in adult sexual relationships. And despite the potential for legal trouble for pedophilic acts, they are driven to child molestation by their own insecurity. For the pedophile, domination and control of a child is sexually stimulating; the pedophile does not have the confidence or ability to manage adult sexual interactions.

The incidence of pedophilic behavior is likely to increase further due to the disintegration of families and the lack of proper supervision of children. But no amount of supervision of children and education about the prevalence of this disorder will eliminate it completely.

Zoophilia

This is the desire to use animals as the main source of sexual stimulation. It usually begins in childhood as a sexual desire for a domestic or farm animal. Whereas this urge may be transient in some children and adolescents, in persons with zoophilia, it is the persistent and preferred way of sexual arousal. This disorder is not common.

Exhibitionism

This is the extreme desire to expose the genitals to a stranger. The act is preferred to normal sexual relationships. When men publicly expose themselves to women, they usually get a frightened and alarmed response. Most women react to the man as though he is about to assault them. However, it is very rare for an exhibitionist to be aggressive and abusive in an overt way. I doubt that there are any exhibitionists who have also been rapists. The reason for this is that men who are exhibitionists are very passive in their relationships with women. The excitement for the man is to see the reaction of alarm in the woman when she sees his genitals exposed. The exhibitionist gains a sense of power by this form of acting out behavior (Goldman, 1988, p. 450).

Recently, I saw a young, married man named Joe, who was referred by his attorney because of a charge of exhibitionism. The man had exhibited himself on a number of occasions but had only been legally accused of the act this time. (Incidently, I have never had an exhibitionist come to me for psychotherapy without a formal charge having preceded the consultation. There appears to be an incredible amount of denial of the existence of the problem until legal concerns enter the person's life.)

Joe had a poor emotional relationship with his wife. Their sexual involvement was also impaired. The patient was very passive in expressing his sexual needs, and his wife did not initiate sexual intercourse. As a Protestant fundamentalist, Joe felt that it was sinful to masturbate, so he did not find this a satisfactory alternative as a sexual outlet. As a result of the unhappy marital relationship, he found himself more and more in need of relating to other women. However, he did not dare to do this within the confines of his marriage; he chose to exhibit himself to young women. Although this created considerable guilt, he was not able to refrain from exhibiting himself repeatedly for several years. Only the fear of a jail sentence was enough to help him suppress his sexual desires long enough to stop his acting out.

I think it is clear that the problem with this patient was one of self-esteem, identity as a man, and the need for an improved relationship with his wife, particularly in the area of assertiveness. These are problems that can respond to psychotherapy in the motivated person. Exhibitionism is the one paraphilia that is most responsive to outpatient psychotherapy.

Sexual Sadism

Persons who engage in sadistic acts are not seen often by psychiatrists, unless the acting-out behavior is distressing to them or they have been legally charged with performing sadistic acts. This condition is probably more common than is generally known.

Sexual sadism is an overwhelming sexual urge to inflict emotional or physical pain on another person whether in fantasy or in reality. The DSM-IV requires that it be present for a period of at least six months to be diagnosed as a disorder. The disorder of sexual sadism is named after the Marquis de Sade, who was known to be cruel and violent toward women.

Just how this trait evolves in the life of humans is not entirely clear. There is now evidence that during childhood one has to be the object of sadistic acts in order to obtain sexual excitement from performing such acts as an adult. Statistically, sexually or physically abused children often become abusive adults. Some psychoanalysts emphasize the pleasure of being aggressive and controlling of others, rather than being controlled by or the object of someone else's sadism. I am struck with the fact that only humans seem to be capable of inflicting pain and suffering in association with the sexual act. To my knowledge, this is unknown in the animal kingdom.

Sexual Masochism

It is equally puzzling that some humans are able to derive pleasure from being injured or humiliated while engaging in sexual acts. Again, this probably does not occur without some similar experience during childhood. Unless the individual feels very upset by these acts, it is unlikely that he or she will come into treatment for the condition.

Sexual masochism is a sexual pleasure accompanied by being harmed either physically or mentally whether in fantasy or in reality. The DSM-IV states that it must be present for at least six months to be considered a disorder. It is the direct opposite of sadism.

In viewing how our patients adapt to life, psychotherapists will sometimes describe someone as having masochistic or sadistic tendencies. For example, if a person allows him or herself to be stepped on frequently in a verbal or interpersonal sense, we say that person is masochistic. In this instance, it is not used in a sexual context. Similarly, there are sadistic people who seem to enjoy making others uncomfortable or embarrassed (always liking to play practical jokes), or worse, by being very critical and verbally abusive. These may be character traits that have little or nothing to do with sexuality. Our language has allowed for such traits to be so described with the terms sadism and masochism. When sadism and masochism become deeply ingrained character traits, they are very hard to treat psychotherapeutically. If the traits are mild and not frequent, there is a greater chance for change.

Voyeurism

Voyeurism is a preference for obtaining sexual arousal by viewing someone naked, undressing, or involved in the sexual act, without the observed person being aware of the voyeur.

According to the DSM-IV, the behavior has to be present for at least six months. It can begin in adolescence or young adult life. Voyeurism is generally accompanied by masturbation for sexual release.

When I first entered private practice over 30 years ago, I had patients who were voyeurs referred to me by lawyers or from the courts. In the last ten years, I have had no such referrals. Meanwhile, I have seen patients with the other paraphilias mentioned. I could not help but wonder why these problems occurred. My speculation is that the sexual freedom that has come about in recent years has enabled voyeurs to go undiscovered, because in our present culture they are able to view any form of pornography at will. I am referring particularly to pornographic videotapes.

Frotteurism

This is a condition is which the man seeks sexual gratification or fantasies from rubbing his penis up against the buttocks of a woman in a public place such as a subway, bus, or other crowded area. The condition is rare. Persons with this disorder do not seek professional help very often.

Atypical Paraphilia

There are a number of unusual and rare paraphilias, about which little is known. The common ingredient is that each produces sexual excitement and may be the preferred method of sexual stimulation. Perhaps the most bizarre is necrophilia–fantasies about sex or sexual activity with a dead body. Others are coprophilia (feces), urophilia (urine), scatologia (obscene phone calls), and mysophilia (dirty surroundings). These conditions are rare with the exception of scatologia. Persons afflicted with these aberrations in sexual preference do not readily admit to having such fantasies or acting-out behaviors.

SEXUAL DYSFUNCTIONS

There are a variety of problems that involve sexual functioning. Only the main disorders will be discussed here. It is assumed that the reader is familiar with the various stages of sexual arousal, which can be read in any basic book about sexual physiology. Treatment of these disorders will be discussed at the end of this section.

Sexual Desire Disorder

There are two types in this group:

1. *Hypoactive sexual desire* is a condition in which the person has few fantasies about sex and little or no desire for sexual activity.

2. *Sexual aversion disorder* is an avoidance of genital contact with a partner for a significant period of time.

Hypoactive sexual disorder may occur at any age in both males and females although reports indicate that it is more common among females. Some affected individuals have a long history of low interest in sexual activity. In others, sexual relations may fade out after a partner becomes ill or disabled. For example, if a man has a heart attack, he may be afraid to resume the physical activity required during sexual contact. Other factors such as guilt, depression, performance anxiety, and anger may prevent a normal interest in sex. In marriage, any sustained disharmony between the couple may result in a decrease in sexual desire, which may become more permanent if the discord continues. Other emotional upsets resulting from major losses due to surgery, financial loss, death of persons that are close, perceived threats to self-esteem, or loss of self-esteem may produce a decrease in sexual desire. Such situations also may occur in stable marriages. Drug abuse and alcoholism may contribute to lack of desire. There also are neurologic, cardiac, and metabolic (diabetes) diseases that lead to decreased or absent sexual desire.

Treatment of this disorder can be done in the context of psychotherapy or using Masters and Johnson's techniques of sexual therapy, which will be described later.

Sexual aversion disorder may be either a severe avoidance of anything involved with sex or a phobic reaction to it with concomitant physical symptoms. The level of intensity of avoidance may vary at different times. It occurs more often in females. There are usually historical reasons for the onset of this disorder–early sexual trauma, overly punitive reactions to early sex play, or excessive reinforcement of guilt.

Sexual Arousal Disorder

There are two conditions included in this classification:

1. Female sexual arousal disorder
2. Male erectile disorder

In these conditions sexual desire is consistently present, but there are problems with sexual arousal.

Female sexual arousal disorder was formerly called frigidity. In this condition, sexual desire may persist, but the woman is not able to be aroused to a state of sexual excitement. Normal vaginal lubrication may not occur, making intercourse difficult.

Male erectile disorder, or impotence, occurs when the male can not have a full penile erection or fails to become erect at all. Among young adult males, about 8 percent are impotent. About 10 to 20 percent of males have some form of erectile difficulty. If a man is able to have early morning erections and also have erections leading to masturbation, then he is presumed to be physically normal. If such a person has problems with erection when coitus is expected, then the problem is obviously psychological in nature. If an organic problem is suspected, then a number of diagnostic tests are available to rule out physical causes, which can be neurologic, circulatory, or metabolic in origin.

In both the male and female disorders, an important reason for the problem is the anxiety about performance. This becomes magnified with failures at subsequent attempts to have sexual relations. Couples often think that their ability to perform sexually should disappear with age, but recent research indicates that many persons remain sexually active in their seventies and eighties. Studies by Kinsey indicate that about 75 percent of men are impotent after age 80.

Orgasmic Disorders

If a woman is completely unable to have an orgasm with coitus or masturbation, it is referred to as anorgasmia. This occurs in about 5 percent of the female population. About 30 percent of women have difficulty achieving an orgasm although they are not totally anorgasmic. Among the causes for this disorder are fear of pregnancy, guilt about sex, a history of sexual abuse in childhood, and many other psychological factors.

Failure to obtain orgasm in males who have no organic disease is not common. It occurs in about 5 percent of men as a primary problem. These men have never been able to have an ejaculation during intercourse, but may be able to have an orgasm during masturbation. Problems with ejaculation also can result from neurologic diseases such as parkinsonism, medications (tranquilizers and anti-hypertensive drugs), and prostate disease.

Premature Ejaculation

In this condition, the male has an ejaculatory experience before or very soon after entering the vagina. It has been estimated that 35 to 40 percent of men treated for sexual dysfunction complain of premature ejaculation. It is generally caused by anxiety about the sexual encounter. Frequently, there is a history of poor early experiences concerning the control of sexual impulses and involving guilt and secrecy.

Sexual Pain Disorders

Dyspareunia causes pain before, during, or after intercourse in a man or woman. It is much more common in women. It may be caused by physical disease and such illnesses must be ruled out. Inflammation, infection, and tumors are common causes and may be responsible for about 15 percent of dyspareunia in women.

Vagismus is a constriction of the outer one-third of the vagina, preventing sexual intercourse. It may be brought on by fear, trauma, rape, the anticipation of pain, pregnancy, or religious inhibitions.

Sexual Dysfunction Due to a General Medical Condition

These disorders may result from conditions such as diabetes, aging, and trauma to the spinal cord. Neurological conditions and vascular abnormalities in males can produce impotency.

TREATMENT

There are several very useful ways to help those suffering from sexual problems. The first is education. It is amazing that in our present society, which appears to be so sophisticated and knowledgeable about sexual matters, so much misinformation exists. The first task of the psychotherapist is to be certain that the distraught person or couple is fully informed about the basic anatomy and physiology of sex. Many are ignorant of what is normal. Some may have obtained inadequate and misleading information in childhood. Others may be inhibited about searching out the current information about sex that is available in any bookstore.

Psychotherapy is one method that has proven to be helpful in solving sexual problems. This is especially true when the person's emotional difficulties are not related to sex directly, but affect the sexual functioning of the individual. For example, when a person is depressed, there is little emotional energy to do anything. Generally, depressed persons have little libido. Excessive anxiety also can interfere with sexual interest. As the psychotherapist helps the individual with these emotional problems, the sexual disturbances may disappear without directly working on them as a specific problem.

As noted, the paraphilias are very difficult to treat. Persons with these disorders seldom come for treatment unless forced to do so by law. But in the area of sexual dysfunctions, there is much that a psychotherapist can do to correct the disturbance.

In 1966, William H. Masters and Virginia E. Johnson published a book titled *The Human Sexual Response.* It was hailed as a basic primer of normal human sexual behavior. Subsequently, they wrote another book on the treatment of sexual dysfunctions, titled *Human Sexual Inadequacy.* In this work, they described a method that they found useful in the treatment of these troublesome problems. When first used, the treatment consisted of a concentrated two-week effort during which the couple spent much of their time in the clinic with the therapists going through education and retraining in sexual matters. The treatment included "sensate focusing," which is an attempt to have each person experience the full sensations of which they are capable. It begins with nonsexual touching of the arms, legs, and trunk to help the persons reexperience sensations that they probably have forgotten. During this period, sexual contact is discouraged. After a full exploration of the nonsexual areas for several days, the couple is instructed to explore the genital areas without having sexual intercourse. Then finally, when both are ready, the sensate focusing leads to the "play" of intercourse.

Much emphasis is placed on the "play" aspect of the sexual relationship. The couple is discouraged from perceiving the sexual encounter as having succeeded or failed. It is viewed as a game that is neither won or lost, but simply enjoyed regardless of the outcome. It is in this framework that the couple enjoy each other best and are likely to have the optimal sexual experience.

Psychotherapists who have adopted this method have found it impractical to have a couple spend two weeks, full time, in this kind of therapy. Several revisions of the method have met with success. I have found that when the Masters and Johnson techniques are used in educating and counseling couples, it can be done on a weekly or semiweekly basis using the same method of sensate focusing. For example, I treated a young couple who were having marital discord because of the wife's failure to have an orgasm. The husband was feeling inadequate as a lover, and his wife was becoming more and more distant from him. Other aspects of their marriage were working well. After about six months of treatment, the relationship had improved significantly, and the wife began to view the sexual experience from a different perspective. She no longer felt that she was a failure; she began to feel sensations that were completely new to her. Then one day she had an orgasm for the first time in her life. The improvement continued and the therapy was concluded. This type of sexual counseling assumes that the couple has no serious emotional problems aside from the emotional disturbances that result from the sexual area. If a serious emotional disorder exists, it should be handled before an attempt is made to treat the sexual problem. All of the sexual dysfunctions mentioned are treatable by the Master's and Johnson technique. This does not include the paraphilias.

OTHER SEXUAL TOPICS

There are several other sexual areas that I would like to discuss. They are not considered diseases and are not classified as such, but they are of considerable concern to the general population and therefore deserve discussion.

Masturbation

The self-stimulation of the genitals begins very early. It occurs in infancy and childhood as an exploratory experience, presumably associated with pleasure. During adolescence, sexual stimulation is associated with or without ejaculatory pleasure or orgasm. According to Alfred Kinsey's research, masturbation is very common, and virtually all men masturbate at some time in their lives. He also found that about 75 percent of women admit to masturbating at one time or another. Yet, the fact of masturbation has created much anxiety in the mind's of individuals because of the guilt and fears surrounding the subject. Masturbation has been said to cause mental illness, physical deformities, and loss of power and strength. None of this has been substantiated, and masturbation is now considered by physicians as a harmless and quite normal endeavor, and it probably has often substituted for serious antisocial acting-out behaviors such as pedophilia or rape.

There is considerable guilt associated with masturbation, particularly in those who are very religious, even if the particular religion to which the person belongs has no specific prohibition against the act. When mental illness occurs and a patient is overly concerned with masturbatory activity, his guilty thoughts can easily lead him to the conclusion that the masturbation caused the illness.

Masturbation is abnormal when it becomes an obsession. Persons so affected may masturbate five to six times a day and cannot refrain from doing so. Such a disturbance should be regarded as another obsessive behavior similar to constant eating, when the eating is done quite aside from hunger or any physical need for sustenance. This form of obsession can be treated by psychotherapy.

Sexual Orientation Distress

Prior to the early part of the 1960s, homosexuality was regarded as a sexual disorder. After that, it was classified as a disorder only if the fact of homosexuality was disturbing to the individual. It was called egodystonic homosexuality. In the present nomenclature in the DSM-IV, it is not mentioned as a separate diagnosis. Under the heading of sexual disorder not otherwise specified, there are three patterns described, one of which is "persistent and marked distress about sexual orientation." Homosexuality is now regarded by the psychiatric community as a variation of normal sexuality. Kinsey reports that about 4 percent of adults are exclusively homosexual, and that 13 percent of the population are predominantly homosexual for at least three years between the ages of 16 to 55. They also report that one in three men have at least one homosexual experience leading to orgasm during postpubertal years. More recent studies have indicated that the prevalence of individuals who are exclusively homosexual is 1 percent of the population. For women, these rates are generally lower than for men (Kaplan and Sadock, 1994, p. 658).

Hormone studies during the prenatal period are of interest. If there is a sufficient amount of male hormone (androgens) in the fetus before birth, it appears to contribute to the heterosexual orientation. If there is a deficiency of male hormone during this period, there is a sexual orientation toward males. Such facts do not prove that there is a hormonal influence in humans that affects how an adult will be oriented sexually, but these studies are provocative and will help to enlighten the confusion in sexual orientation (Kaplan and Sadock, 1994, p. 659).

In studies of twins the concordance toward homosexuality is greater than in normal siblings. That is, if one twin is homosexual, it is more likely that the other twin also will be oriented in this direction. Some families show a higher rate of homosexuality than the rest of the population, indicating the possibility of genetic factors. Much more research will be required to clarify this matter.

Sexuality is very diverse and complicated. It can cause much distress in the physical and emotional aspects of life. The ethical concerns of society regarding sexual matters have become diluted almost to the point of nonexistence. Psychotherapists certainly have not been leaders in the field of morality. It has been the clergy who have been consistently speaking to these matters. But as time goes on, it becomes more and more confusing to each new generation. Values change as society views sex in different ways. For example, recently the New York Board of Regents ruled that it would be prudent to have condoms available to the adolescent population in public schools in order to prevent the spread of AIDS. This would have been unthinkable even 20 years ago.

Many are questioning the message being given to our youth, when it is implied by educational authorities that sexual relations are permitted as long as the adolescent avoids disease. What are the moral implications of such behavior on the developing child, and what effect will this have on the future of the family? I suspect it will have devastating results. Unrestricted sexual activity does not appear to have helped society, nor has it reduced sexual acting out in the form of rape and paraphiliac behavior or the degree to which the public suffers from neurosis. As noted, with increased sexual freedom, new problems have evolved, but society does not appear to be any more at peace with itself.

WHAT CAN THE CLERGY DO?

1. When sexual difficulties occur in marriage, it is often due to trouble in the relationship. Prudent attention to the problems in the marriage and help in resolving issues will often result in the sexual difficulty improving. Clergy who become skilled in marriage counseling can be of help in this area.
2. If you do not feel competent to deal with marriage problems or if one or both of your married congregants is suffering from a sexual disorder, you may feel that you are in over your head in knowing what to do to help. Do not be afraid to ask for assistance from a competent marriage counselor.
3. Persons suffering from a paraphilia usually do not seek treatment, nor are they readily responsive to treatment, except in the case of exhibitionism. Research is being done in this area. There is hope that some of the newer antidepressants may be helpful in these conditions. If you are aware that one of your congregants has a paraphilia, refer him or her to a psychotherapist who is familiar with these disorders. Your intervention may be an important step in helping the affected person begin controlling the sexual problem. You may also help him or her in avoiding legal difficulties.
4. To some extent, sexual urges, whether abnormal or not, can be modified or controlled by spiritual means via prayer and meditation. But it is important that the clergy be realistic and not naive in assessing their own abilities in this area.
5. There is one other condition that is mentioned in textbooks, about which the clergy should know. It has no official diagnosis. It is called pseudohomosexual anxiety. In this condition, the young adult wrongly assumes that he is homosexual and

becomes very anxious about it. He may draw this conclusion from the fact that he is not having sex with women like his male friends are. Sometimes, he may not feel as driven toward sexuality as others, or he may have had one or more homosexual dreams or fantasies. Whatever the reason, it is important to help such a person to appreciate his true sexual orientation. If his *predominant* sexual drive is toward the opposite sex, then you can assure him that he is heterosexual. An occasional homosexual thought or fantasy does not mean that the person is oriented in that direction. Again, if you are unsure of yourself in this area, consult with a psychotherapist in whom you have confidence.

6. Guilt and sexuality are often linked together. Here the clergy should differentiate between true guilt and neurotic or psychotic guilt. True guilt must be assessed and handled in the religious context of the congregant with his clergyperson. Abnormal guilt usually does not respond to the exhortations and rituals that the clergy can offer. When your usual ministrations do not relieve the guilt of the distressed person, be suspect that you may be dealing with a guilt that is abnormal. A competent psychotherapist can handle such guilt in terms of its origin, nature (psychotic or neurotic), and how it is linked to other factors in the person's life. While not always easy to treat, there is hope for the person suffering from the burden of abnormal guilt feelings.

Chapter 13

Eating Disorders

You have heard it said: "You are what you eat." Nutritionists like to use this statement to emphasize that eating can influence how you feel in terms of energy, enthusiasm, and the general feeling of well-being. I agree that it matters that we watch our diet, eat well, stay trim, and not abuse our bodies. But all of us are aware that we are also very much influenced by what we think. The cognitive psychotherapists are impressed with the tremendous effect that our daily thoughts have on our feelings and behavior. To me, there is no doubt that our thoughts greatly influence how we react to events. And, of course, the appropriate use of our feelings—our emotions—also contributes much to our general feeling of health.

What you eat, think, and feel are factors in how your day proceeds. In addition, if your body is in pain or an illness is present, it complicates matters even more.

In this chapter I will discuss the eating disorders. Before doing so, let us start where it all begins.

EARLY FEEDING

The pregnant mother feeds the developing fetus via the umbilical cord. When normal birth occurs, oral feeding begins. If you touch an infant's cheek, it will turn its head in the direction of the touch. This is called the rooting reflex. The newborn is looking for the source of food via an instinctual reflex to feed. The sucking reflex is another normal response of the infant to the need for nourishment.

The interaction between the child and the mother is important in developing a calm, unhurried response to eating, as opposed to a tense, anxiety-filled experience. Psychiatrists, such as Harry Stack Sullivan, maintained that the early interaction between mother and child was the beginning of the road to mental health or illness. It was his opinion that if the mother was anxious, it created anxiety in the child, leading to later feelings of estrangement from the mother.

Of course, parental attitudes toward eating are important. When the developing child does not eat well for several weeks, it does not mean that there is a serious problem. Children go through various stages of eating a little or a lot. This should not be taken as a foreboding signal. The important thing is the child's overall development within the range of expected norms, rather than what happens on a given day or week.

Some parents become alarmed when a child does not eat all of her food. Forcing a child to eat food that she may not need or finds distasteful really can help no one. Parental obsessions with nutrition often result in arguments at the dinner table. Such a situation certainly cannot be good for mental health or nutrition. I have long believed that the emotional battles at the dinner table probably contribute more to the stress of growing up than does conflict over bowel training or even early sexual development. It is amazing how few studies have been done on the interaction of parent and child in the area of feeding and the subsequent neurotic trends that follow.

AN OVERVIEW OF EATING DISORDERS

Although there are other disorders in the classification, the problems that we see most in the clinical setting are anorexia, bulimia, and obesity. The latter is not formerly included in the DSM-IV although it is generally considered a disorder that causes considerable emotional and physical harm.

Obesity may be brought on, consciously or unconsciously, by the fear of sexuality and the fear of being attractive to the opposite sex. Some women test the sincerity of men by being obese, to see if the man is attracted to their mind or personality rather than their body. Men sometimes enjoy being obese as they associate obesity with strength and power.

Many studies reveal evidence that the emotional relationships in a family can bring on the serious conditions of anorexia (loss of at least 15 percent of ideal body weight), bulimia (binge eating followed by purging), or obesity. Generally speaking, the attitude of children toward eating is affected by at least three factors:

1. Parental attitudes toward food
2. Peer pressure about what, how, and when to eat
3. Cultural fads, such as what is advertised on TV, the latest styles in dress, the size and shape of models, and health fads

There is some evidence that parents can overfeed their children and thus create obesity, which can persist into adult life. Some parents are charter members of the "clean plate club." They act as though the very life of the child depends on what happens at each meal. And, of course, parents become instant sociologists when they remind their offspring, "There are children all over the world starving to death, and you won't eat your dinner." If a parent's attitude is severe in the area of eating, the child often develops a negative reaction to suggestions that are made.

Peer pressure regarding eating habits needs little explanation. This applies equally to dress codes, styles, and fashions of youth, all of which affect eating habits. Titian models are simply not in fashion today. The figure of Twiggy was quite undesirable a few centuries ago, or even 50 years ago. In some cultures, it is still not popular, and the full-figured woman is much preferred.

When I was in medical school, the condition of anorexia nervosa was mentioned as a rare but important disease. During my eight years of medical school, internship, and residency training, I saw only one case of anorexia. In the intervening years, this disease has become an epidemic.

Bulimia was hardly ever discussed in the past. Now some college campuses claim that as many as 25 to 30 percent of their female students practice binge eating and purging at some time in their college careers.

When I started my private practice, I encountered a 17-year-old female patient who admitted to me that each night she dutifully ate all her dinner ("cleaned the plate") to satisfy her mother. However, she then went into the bathroom and vomited her meal to satisfy herself; she wanted to stay slim. It was the early 1960s; I had as yet not heard of bulimia.

Bulimia and anorexia are rare among men, although the incidence is increasing of late. Thus far, these illnesses are not seen much in the inner city populations. They are manifested more often in the middle and upper-middle classes. The opposite can be said for obesity, which appears to be more common among lower-class families. One can speculate on the reasons for this class difference. To my knowledge, no scientific studies have been done in this area.

In obesity and anorexia there is a distortion of body image. The person simply does not see his or her physical body as others see it. The anorexic, who can appear like a concentration camp victim, looks into the mirror and sees "fat." The obese person does not "see" the obesity to the extent that it exists. The expression "fat and happy" implies an indulgence with food but also a certain denial of the obese condition.

In order to appreciate disturbances of body image, consider the normal distortions that occur to all of us. My friend says that when he looks into the mirror, he sees that he has a full head of hair. Only a photograph of himself shows the truth of his marked balding. Similar distortions occur with aging. When I was much younger, a 60-year-old patient told me that his mind and feelings told him that he was no more than 35 or 40. I found this hard to believe. But, now that I have passed 60 myself, I marvel at his insight. In effect, the psyche fails to keep up with the aging of the body. The psychic representation of ourselves remains younger than our age. This sometimes leads us to do things only a younger person would do.

A more dramatic example of this is found in the condition called "phantom limb." In this case, a person has had an amputation of his leg, and for as long as a year, he continues to feel pain or itching in his missing foot. Apparently, the psychic representation of his foot and the remembered sensations remain in the brain for a long time in spite of the missing limb.

On a lesser note, although physical limitations have reminded me of the reality of aging, I still think of myself as a young athlete. This idea is momentarily reinforced while skiing and playing tennis. I have moments of fantasy when I am "poetry in motion" on the slope or court—just about ready for the Olympics. Of course, this is usually followed abruptly by missed moguls or miss-hit tennis balls. Our minds are capable of great distortions of reality in many dimensions of living. The area of eating is no exception. And no wonder! It is such an important drive: our very life depends on it.

Classification of Eating Disorders

The DSM-IV of the American Psychiatric Association lists two eating disorders in adults:

1. Anorexia nervosa
2. Bulimia

As noted, the DSM-IV does not list obesity as a specific eating disorder. But, since obesity is such a serious health issue, I will discuss it in detail as well. When psychological factors are regarded as important in the origin of obesity, the illness is classified under Psychological Factors Affecting Medical Condition.

ANOREXIA NERVOSA

Mary was 14 years old but could easily have passed for 12. She was severely anorexic and weighed 75 pounds. Her physician was concerned that she would continue to lose weight and be in danger of dying.

Mary had her rituals about food. She was very compulsive, ate exactly on schedule, but only enough to prevent herself from losing more weight. She appeared depressed, had little to say, and seemed like a lost soul. Prior to her illness, she had many friends and was popular. Her academic work was superior, and she had a keen interest in sports and other school activities. But now there was a deterioration in all areas.

The daily routine included weighing herself and looking in the mirror. Fat was a revolting sight to her, and she saw it all over her body when she viewed herself in the mirror. Even photographs of herself in a bathing suit did not convince her that she was excessively thin.

In addition to the physical problems, Mary was always upset. Although usually quiet, she had periods of anger and rage that her parents had never seen before. These outbursts were followed by childlike crying that made her parents cuddle her like a two-year-old. Incidently, I have seen nothing scare parents more that anorexia, not even drug abuse. As one mother put it, "You just have no control over what your child does to herself. It's frightening to think that you can do nothing to stop your child's behavior." Watching a child starve herself to death runs so contrary to the primitive instinct to feed and to nourish.

Mary had considerable difficulty talking about her problem. She was not naturally verbal, and at times it was easier to get her to write about her emotions than to talk about them. When she was alone with me, she was not able to speak adequately about her feelings toward her parents and siblings. In family sessions, with her mother's encouragement, she expressed her feelings better.

Because of the profound weight loss that Mary had experienced, hospitalization was considered. Mary did not want to leave home, and her parents wanted to attempt caring for her there.

I saw Mary several times a week in my office, and gave her an antidepressant to both help her mood and her appetite. In spite of the fact that she was unable to resolve her emotional problems fully, she did gain weight and in about nine months was back to a satisfactory level. Mary was not as motivated toward therapy as I had hoped she would be, so I elected to talk to her parents in subsequent sessions to help them resolve their conflicts regarding Mary and her anorexia.

Generally, if the patient is older and more verbal, there is a better chance of establishing a therapeutic relationship that can uncover the salient intrapsychic problems as well as family-related issues. Sometimes family therapy is the most effective method that can be utilized. Hospitalization with behavior modification may be necessary and may be lifesaving.

What kind of illness can bring about such a life-threatening condition in young people? How can a young girl starve herself in the presence of adequate food and parents who are concerned? There are no easy answers to these questions.

If ever there was a disease of affluence, it is anorexia. It is rare in the ghetto, among the poor, and in less-developed countries. It has come into vogue in the last two generations. The occurence of anorexia is five times higher in females than males. It begins in early adolescence and can continue well into adult life. By definition, the diagnosis is made if the person is not suffering from another disease and has lost 15 percent of his or her baseline (ideal) weight. Most anorexics lose much more than 15 percent. At one time I saw an adolescent who weighed 55 pounds. When reaching such extremes of weight loss, the body is losing muscle tissue and the patient is close to death.

Anorexia is characterized by an obsession with food and hoarding of food. Most anorexics are very compulsive and ritualistic in food preparation and their personal habits. In order to control weight, they use diet pills and laxatives; sometimes they vomit or engage in severe exercise routines to lose weight.

In addition, patients suffering from this malady are often depressed and sometimes suicidal. They may have a variety of physical disorders, such as abdominal distress, amenorrhea (cessation of menstrual periods), excessive hair growth on arms and legs, and cardiac problems. In males, there is a low testosterone level. Among females, estrogen levels are decreased, and other endocrine disorders occur, including thyroid disturbances.

Anorexia can begin at or around puberty and at different stages of development. It can begin with such changes as starting high school or college or after tragedies in the person's life. It can present as a single episode or become chronic. Death may occur because of malnutrition. Some studies show death occurring in as much as 20 percent of cases. The suicide rate runs as high as 5 percent.

Anorexia often occurs after severe dieting. It has been observed in ballet dancers, jockeys, gymnasts, and wrestlers, all of whom are concerned with weight control. A biological vulnerability to continued anorexia appears to follow such severe weight control.

Psychological and Behavioral Problems

The typical adolescent anorexic patient is striving for independence while still remaining very dependent on the family. There is often a fierce rejection of parents, while internally the patient is feeling very inadequate and dependent.

Body image is affected severely. Anorexics simply do not see themselves as others see them. They look in the mirror and see fat everywhere on their bodies.

In their attempt to control, they think in all-or-nothing terms. On any given day a parent is the most wonderful parent in the world, and the next day, the worst excuse for a parent that a person could ever have. When in the hospital, they tend to polarize the staff into good and bad persons. Those suffering from anorexia have a deep need to control not only food, weight, and their appearance, but also the significant people around them.

Among the possible causes of this serious disorder are the following:

1. The cultural emphasis on being thin was not a factor 50 years ago, and the phenomenon of anorexia was uncommon. As styles change in the future, it is possible that one day the "thin" look may no longer be sought after, and there could be a rapid decline in the disease.

2. In some anorexics there is clearly an attempt to avoid sexuality and the changes and responsibilities of growing up. There is the desire, usually unconscious, to remain the prepubescent little boy or girl, who can be taken care of by her parents.

3. There is often a problem of separation from parental figures. While still wanting to remain abnormally dependent, the person still correspondingly desires to be independent. This problem of individuation begins at a very early age, and the child may have had difficulty dealing with this process for many years.

4. Most authorities in the field are impressed with the fact that the families of anorexic patients are dysfunctional in a number of ways, which differs with every family. Basically it appears that the families do not provide the proper climate in which the developing child can comfortably grow and develop and separate from the parents at the appropriate stages.

Treatment of Anorexia

The first problem that must be dealt with in treating anorexia is the matter of nutrition. This is usually done by a physician or nutritionist who can monitor weight gain and food intake. The goal here is to return the person to normal eating habits. Someone other than the psychotherapist should be in control of the patient's diet. It is almost impossible to be a watchdog and disciplinarian about nutrition and a psychotherapist at the same time.

In hospital settings the food intake is monitored often in conjunction with behavioral modification techniques using operant conditioning. Rewards and privileges are given for weight gain and good food intake. Patients are watched for manipulative behavior such as purging, using laxatives, and exercising excessively to lose weight. One nurse is assigned to be the disciplinarian and thereby assumes the "bad guy" role, while another nurse plays the role of psychotherapist. The latter is looked on as the "good guy" in the eyes of the anorexic patient. In addition to behavioral therapy, individual, group, and family therapy are all useful in helping the anorexic develop a sense of autonomy and self-esteem. The separation-individuation problems and the all-or-nothing thinking are important issues to clarify with the patient.

Medications can also be useful in the treatment of anorexia. The antidepressants (Tofranil, Elavil, Nardil) help with the patient's depression. Neuroleptics (Thorazine, Haldol, Navane, Mellaril) in low doses relieve anxiety. Both categories of drugs have an effect on weight gain by changing the patient's metabolism. The mechanism for this phenomenon is not understood.

Recently, support groups have been formed throughout the country to assist anorexic patients and their families. These are low-cost groups that try to educate and counsel anyone who is suffering from anorexia. Some find these groups of enormous value, particularly after the acute phase of the disease is past.

BULIMIA

This illness was first described in the late 1950s. It consists of binge eating large amounts of food over a short amount of time. It may occur in those of normal weight or in obese or anorexic individuals. The binge eating may happen even though the person is not hungry. Rather, it appears to be a response to emotional needs, to relieve anxiety, depression, loneliness, or other uncomfortable states. Some patients binge and purge many times a day while others do so as infrequently as weekly or less often. While many bulimics purge after binge eating, some prefer to fast instead of purging. Binge eating is generally not a public ritual, but is done privately; it is not a behavior that one talks about freely to others. On occasion, bulimics have been known to drink excessively, steal, and exhibit suicidal behavior.

According to some reports, normal-weight bulimics appear confused about hunger; they stay hungry even after eating a sufficient amount. Bulimics also use calories more efficiently than normal persons.

Mild forms of bulimia are common. Many college students are affected by this disorder. Some learn how to binge and purge from peers in the same way that the young learn to drink and take drugs. It seems to be a quasi-acceptable form of behavior, and there appears to be little peer pressure to stop the behavior.

A 19-year-old woman came to me for consultation for bulimia at the request of her parents. She was in no great distress, but she admitted that her infrequent binge eating and purging disgusted her. She was aware of her need to control her weight in this manner. As yet, the bulimia had not adversely affected her physically. She was gradually able to stop the process and watch her diet in a more normal way.

In contrast, another patient had a severe case of bulimia that was causing great distress. She had ulcers in her esophagus and mouth. The enamel in her teeth had begun to disappear, and at times she became dehydrated and had a serum electrolyte imbalance. This latter condition can be very serious and result in cardiac problems and even death if not treated in a hospital.

People suffering from severe bulimia do an incredible amount of eating during the binge eating periods. The copious consumption of food may temporarily satisfy an inner craving. One can speculate on what this hunger is about. Certainly it involves the appetite for food, but psychologically it speaks of other needs as well. Some experts in this field refer to unfulfilled sexual needs or fears of sexual involvement. Others point to the need for security represented in food and in the act of eating. Still others feel that the image of the slender youthful figure is of paramount importance, at least on a conscious level. There is also the act of eating to satisfy the external and internalized parental figures, while pleasing the self by vomiting and staying slim. Since most persons suffering from bulimia have low self-esteem, it has been theorized that they are attempting unconsciously to expel in a symbolic manner unwanted parts of the self (Kaplan, Sadock, and Grebb, 1994, pp. 695, 697).

As with all such theories, one has to understand the patient thoroughly in order to ferret out what psychological problems are present in any particular case.

Treatment of Bulimia

It is important that treatment of this disorder begin early in the course of the disease. At the beginning, if the pattern has not yet become habitual, it may be easier to stop. When the binge eating and purging have gone on for years and have become an established life pattern, it is much harder to interrupt.

Psychotherapy is regarded as the treatment of choice for bulimia, with or without the use of behavior modification. Support groups for persons with bulimia are helpful, especially if the group consists of peers. Various antidepressants have been used for bulimia when the patient has concomitant depression. The antidepressant Prozac appears to be effective in helping bulimia in about 60 percent of cases.

OBESITY

It is assumed by the general public that obesity is simply a matter of excessive caloric intake. However, the research that has been done indicates that it is not simply due to overeating. It appears to be a combination of genetic, metabolic, psychosocial, and central nervous system functions although these factors are not understood very well. Even the use of calories obtained from different sources do not appear to be identical as formerly thought; 1,000 calories contained in a dessert are not identical to 1,000 calories obtained from vegetables as far as the utilization in the body is concerned.

By definition, obesity is present when an individual is at least 20 percent above ideal weight. The latter is not well standardized, since it varies somewhat from one culture to another. By the 20 percent standard, there are many people in our society who are obese. The prevalence of obesity among adults in the United States has been estimated as 15 percent to 50 percent. It is more common in women and as people age.

Obesity is more frequent in first-generation ethnic groups in this country and in lower socioeconomic groups. It is known to be higher in particular ethnic groups such as Hungarians, Czechoslovakians, Italians, and the British. Also, obesity is higher among Jews, less among Catholics, and least among Protestants (Goldman, 1988, p. 465).

There is good evidence that heredity plays a part. If one parent is obese, there is a 40 percent chance that the adolescent children will be obese. If both parents are obese, the figure rises to 80 percent. Although environmental influences are important in the prevalence of obesity, adopted children raised by obese parents generally do not have a high rate of obesity. This favors the theory of genetic predisposition.

Metabolic factors also play a part. It is well-known that persons with hypothyroidism tend to become obese. There are rare endocrine disorders that also cause obesity.

Although symptoms such as anxiety, depression, and guilt are often associated with obesity, there is no evidence that a specific personality type is more likely to be obese. One interesting theory states that the obese individual reacts to the sight and smells of food more than others, and therefore eats more often and eats greater quantities. The naturally slender person tends to be less influenced by these factors and is more likely to eat when he is hungry.

Physiological Theories of Obesity

In recent years the set-point theory has been studied. It states that if an individual eats excessively or diets strenuously, the person eventually will return to approximately the same weight. Animal experiments strongly support this theory, but it is more difficult to demonstrate this in humans. After dieting, most people find it very difficult to maintain their weight at the desired level and will return to their set point—a return to the former weight after an interval of time. However, the opposite is not true. Those who gain weight and become obese do not easily return to a set point as animals are likely to do.

There is also the fat-cell theory. There is good evidence that fat cells accumulate in the body at two specific times–before age 2 and again from ages 10 to 14. Once formed these fat cells do not disappear. They may become larger or smaller, but their number remains the same. Those individuals who have a large number of fat cells from childhood are more likely to be obese (Goldman, 1988, p. 465).

Other factors that control eating are the appetite center located in the lower part of the brain, neurotransmitters that carry messages in the brain, gastrointestinal hormones, a variety of diseases such as cancer, and many other internal and external influences.

Psychological Theories of Obesity

Early psychoanalytical ideas begun by Freud indicated that obesity was due to unresolved dependency needs and was due to a fixation at the oral level of psychological development. Some obese persons do have an unusual preoccupation with food, much as the alcoholic is consumed with obtaining and drinking alcohol. But recent studies do not show an increase in psychological disorders in obese individuals as compared to the normal population. Some obese persons suffer from a negative self-concept and feel rejected by others. A small subgroup has a distorted body image. But these changes appear to be the result of obesity rather than the cause of it.

In some families, parents feed their children excessively, equating food with love. In some societies, food is a symbol of prosperity. In our country, thinness is of greater concern in the middle class or upper class, in which the quantity of food is stressed less than the quality.

Physiological Result of Obesity

There are diseases that are caused by or aggravated by obesity. High blood pressure and heart disease, with an increase in serum cholesterol and triglycerides, are commonly associated with obesity. The hyperinsulinism (with low blood sugar) common in obese persons may eventually lead to diabetes. In women, menstrual irregularities, polycystic kidneys, and abnormal hair growth can occur. In men, decreased libido and impotence are common. Shortness of breath, osteoarthritis, gouty arthritis, and an increased incidence of gallstones are all associated with obesity.

The Treatment of Obesity

There are a number of approaches to the problem of obesity, none of which is guaranteed to succeed in permanently changing the obesity unless the dieter is willing to exercise consistent effort. Consuming fewer calories has been the mainstay of diet programs. Food substitutes in liquid form are common. More recently calories have been less emphasized. Rather, a decreased intake of fat has been recommended by nutritionists. A low-fat diet appears to be more important in terms of health than the obsession with caloric intake. Foods such as pasta, which is low in fat but higher in calories than vegetables, has been recommended.

Medicines that reduce appetite are still used but are not very effective in consistently reducing the desire to eat. If someone has an enormous appetite and always feels hungry, the medications may be beneficial. Tenuate and Pondimin are among the safest and most prescribed. The use of medications without dieting has little effect. Some patients find it helpful to have an appetite suppressant to help them start dieting.

In the last decade, exercise has been recommended as helpful in losing weight because it increases metabolism and decreases appetite. While this statement has validity, exercise is known to be more helpful in prevention of weight gain than in losing weight. To be effective in weight prevention or in association with dieting, exercise has to be repeated at least three times a week, for 30 minutes and be maintained at this frequency; it should become a lifestyle change.

Behavior modification and hypnotism have been used to treat obesity by trained practitioners of these techniques. In certain individuals these methods may assist in dieting, when the person is unable to obtain results with dieting alone. The organization Weight Watchers is quite successful in using group dynamics and behavior modification techniques in assisting the obese with dieting. Overeaters Anonymous accomplishes similar results by applying the 12-step program of Alcoholics Anonymous. There are some studies that have appeared in the literature that indicate that psychoanalytically oriented psychotherapy has been useful in treating obesity especially in persons with disturbed body image or those with low self-esteem. For those unfortunate individuals who are morbidly obese, surgery is often recommended. Abdominal bypass operations and gastric stapling have been done in order to allow less food to pass into the gastrointestinal tract or allow less food to be absorbed. This type of surgery is not without its dangers, and should be done only by physicians who have had considerable experience with these procedures.

Losing weight may not be the most difficult thing to do. Many people do it often. But how many are able to maintain their weight loss? Statistics say about 10 percent. That is not a very large number.

I think my physician friend, John, has found the answer, although it is not simple. Several years ago he lost 100 pounds. He had been grossly overweight, and he knew that it was affecting his health and ability to function. About a year after he lost the weight, I saw him at a meeting. He had not gained anything in the interim. When I asked him how he accomplished this feat, he said that he basically changed his habits. He eats three meals a day instead of skipping one or two as many people do. He eats much less at each meal and tries to think of eating as a necessity—a requirement to stay alive—rather than a time to indulge his appetite and gorge himself. He also tries to make other parts of his life more interesting; he spends more time reading, listening to music, and pursuing other interests.

John told me that his mother had forced food on him and made him believe that eating was the most important part of the day. John is trying to make it a necessary but relatively unimportant part of his day. He is succeeding!

WHAT THE CLERGY CAN DO

As with other illnesses, the clergy can be very supportive in assisting their congregants in recognizing eating problems, making the proper referrals, and in giving the necessary encouragement required for long-term change.

Families coping with severe eating problems are families that are under great stress. I am not convinced that every such family is dysfunctional in a gross way. But if a child is anorexic or bulimic, the stress on the family is enormous. Hardly anything bothers parents more than the feeling of helplessness that accompanies a child's refusal to eat. The clergy can be very helpful in providing a listening ear to the parents. By doing so, the stress level can be diminished. In crisis situations, the clergy may be asked for direct intervention with the ill child. Here the clergy can be of great assistance in guiding the family to the proper therapeutic setting.

With eating disorders, there is considerable denial of the illness. This is especially true of anorexia and bulimia. Confronting the person with his denial may be a lifesaving act. These illnesses are potentially fatal and therefore should be handled by persons expert in the field. The clergy can be very helpful by taking an active role in bringing these individuals to the proper treatment setting. It is not appropriate for members of the clergy to directly counsel an anorexic child in an attempt to talk him or her into eating.

The obese person usually is not suffering from a critical or life-threatening problem. The clergy may be quite helpful by encouraging the proper nutrition and exercise for the affected person. If a good, trusting relationship prevails between a clergyperson and a congregant, some counseling that focuses on these areas is very useful.

Of course, if a person with an eating disorder has a spiritual problem, the problem should be handled in the usual clerical manner in conjunction with the treating therapist.

Chapter 14

Understanding Stress

There are days when you hear so much about stress, you would think that it was a new discovery. But stress has been known to all living creatures from time immemorial. Remember the last time you were frightened? Like a scared cat, you could feel the hair stand up on your head and your heart pound. You were ready for a fight-or-flight reaction.

But the phenomenon we now call stress has not been called that for very long. It is a concept derived from physics, in which it refers to the physical energy placed on objects such as bridges and airplane wings. But, in human terms, we speak of the effects of stress on the individual more than about the stress itself. We are concerned with poorly handled stress and about symptoms such as anxiety, depression, or psychosomatic reactions.

Basically, stress is a disturbance in equilibrium that requires adjustment. It is a term that was used by the researcher and physiologist Hans Selye in referring to the effect of our environment on the endocrine system. On the basis of his research, he concluded that when a person is stressed, she experiences a reaction in the area of the brain called the hypothalamus, which in turn sends impulses to the pituitary, thyroid, and adrenal glands. This reaction enables the person to cope with the stresses that she encounters. When the stress is perceived as a danger, it results in a fight-or-flight reaction. Such reactions are necessary for survival even today, although to a lesser extent than in the past.

However, there are certain stressors we encounter that are not perceived as danger, but are felt as energizing and pleasant, as in playing a strenuous game of tennis. In some sports, such as skiing and mountain climbing, there is some danger, but it is experienced by those engaging in it as mild stress, and the participant matches her skill and physical ability against the potential danger. The result is mentally and physically rewarding.

In our modern world, we cannot run away from all stress, nor can we physically fight whenever we are stressed. People handle stress in many ways—emotionally as well as physically. Often, our bodies react to that stress which is perceived as danger by developing psychosomatic symptoms such as severe headaches, stomach ulcers, colitis, or other illnesses associated with stress. By becoming physically ill, the person can gracefully back away from a fight—emotional or physical—while not being seen by others as running away. It is our modern-day equivalent of saving face.

We do not always react physically to stress; often our reaction is emotional. When this occurs, our minds use defense mechanisms to deal with stress. For example, the defense of denial is an unconscious way of acting as though the stressor is not present. This is seen especially in alcoholism or in the newly diagnosed cancer patient. Here the person denies that the illness exists or that it is serious and requires attention.

Stress differs for each individual. For some, the act of flying in an airplane is very stressful, but to the commercial airline pilot, flying is "just another day at the office." I have known military men who, when under tension from some stressor, go to an area where paratroopers are jumping. They join the group, and after a jump or two, they feel very relaxed. The parachute jump apparently stresses them in a way that is both stimulating and relaxing. (Somehow, I find it hard to recommend this to my patients as a common remedy for stress.)

More than one person has asked me how I, as a psychiatrist, could possibly tolerate listening to patients hour after hour, the implication being that it is extremely stressful. Although every job has its stressful moments, the practice of psychiatry is probably no more stressful than any other job with a lot of responsibility. I can think of many vocations that I would regard as more stressful than being a psychiatrist—for example, being a member of the clergy or managing billion-dollar portfolios for others.

STRESS: YESTERDAY AND TODAY

For centuries, much of the stress on the individual involved concerns about day-to-day survival. It required physical strength and endurance. The need for our attention to survival has been remarkably reduced by modern industrial development.

We no longer have to walk two miles for a pail of water or cut down trees for firewood or building materials, except if we choose to. Our bodies are not primarily constructed for office work and cognitive jobs. Physically, we have the potential for primitive hunting, fishing, and agriculture, but no longer are we required to use our physical strength to the same degree that was needed by our forefathers. In developed countries, the average person does not have to till the soil or search for food.

Life has become easier and paradoxically more complicated. The stressors of today are very different from the largely agrarian society of the past. Today most of our stresses are mental and emotional, rather than physical. Only the well-trained athlete and those who do daily manual work are in any kind of physical shape to cope with the stresses that were required in previous centuries.

While historical alterations have occurred, our bodies have not kept up with the change. When confronted with stress, we cannot work it off physically as in the past unless we remember to do this through regular exercise. It has taken almost a century for our society to realize that exercise may be necessary for good mental and physical health. Before the turn of the century, most people were moving about by either walking or riding horses or bicycles. Then, new modes of transportation, such as automobiles and buses, transformed all of that, while physically we have remained much the same. Our endocrine systems have not become accustomed to the alteration in habits. The result is that stress appears to be felt much more in physical symptoms and in emotional disturbances since it is not being relieved through natural physiological means with exercise.

There have been many other modifications in our society that have produced stress on our emotional lives. In recent years, everything has evolved more rapidly and changes in society have occurred quickly. It has been estimated that one-fourth of the population relocates each year. This is in marked contrast to the lack of movement from one place to another only 100 years ago.

The media, meanwhile, has assaulted our senses creating further stress. Television has given us pleasure as well as much information, but it has also highlighted our inadequacies and created needs in us that we did not know we had. It has shown us violence and sexual material that we never thought would be shown in our homes. The language used on TV has deteriorated to the lowest level. Recent situation comedies have reached a new low in prurient interests and in general vulgarity. The new-age comedians seem to be stuck in a gutter of four letter words which appear to have become obligatory in the field of comedy.

Children in the suburbs are overly organized while in the large cities there is little direction for children. Where the young children are too rigidly supervised, the adolescents are too free to do as they please. College students lack any supervision at all when most of them would welcome more controls. The prolonged adolescence of the present generation comes with enormous freedom that the average teenager finds baffling–and very stressful.

Some are of the opinion that the young have an easy life, but it is my considered judgment that the young are far more stressed than in the past with many more decisions regarding vocation, sexual choices, and identity concerns. The marked increase in the suicide rate among the young gives evidence to the greater stress that is present.

Meanwhile, institutions have been demythologized, religions have been degraded, schools have been criticized, and we look in vain for role models in our culture that will help our children. Things constantly change; little is predictable. Today's hero is tomorrow's forgotten personality. New is good; old is history. With all this happening, it is surprising that a fair number of children grow up with a minimum of effects from stress.

These rapid changes have resulted in an increase in stress. We are hardly able to overcome one stress before we are faced with two others. Is it any wonder that the increase in emotional problems has required more counseling, and that there has been a proliferation of self-help groups?

HUMAN DEVELOPMENT AND STRESS

We know little of the stress on the fetus that occurs during pregnancy although research is being conducted in this area. It is already clear that the excessive consumption of alcohol by the mother can produce fetal alcohol syndrome. Pregnant women are now warned not to drink alcohol at all to prevent any adverse effect on the developing fetus. The cigarette-smoking mother has been shown to produce babies that are generally of lower weight. A deficiency of vitamins and poor nutrition in the pregnant mother is also known to have ill effects on the fetus. At this point, little is known about how the effects of emotional stress and strain on the mother relates to the developing fetus.

STRESSES OF CHILDHOOD

A great deal of research is being conducted with infants concerning the effects of early environment on physical growth and emotional well-being. Pediatricians have emphasized the need for "bonding" of parents to the newborn child. Only a few short years ago, it was virtually unknown for a new father to enter a delivery room. Now it is commonplace. But, as with all new trends, some individuals overdo what is recommended. I know of a case where the new parents would not allow friends or relatives to visit their home for months because the parents were "bonding" with their new baby. While trying to remedy one problem, we humans frequently create another.

Recently, there has been a trend to have deliveries in the parental home. It remains to be seen whether this will prove to be a permanent trend.

There is little doubt that a close relationship of the mother to the infant is a necessary and positive experience for the infant. The importance of this relationship was emphasized by the American psychiatrist Harry Stack Sullivan. It was his opinion that basic anxiety begins with the anxious mother transferring her anxiety to the child, who then becomes insecure about obtaining basic needs. This occurs when the mother is highly neurotic, psychotic, or has a personality that interferes with adequate mothering. In such instances, the child would be cared for better by a substitute mother. Although this may be true, it is not easy for any society to enforce alternate or substitute mothering.

In today's environment there is considerably more childcare done by baby-sitters than ever before. We hear so much about child abuse that one wonders whether this is not bordering on hysteria, played up by the media. There seems to be little doubt, however, that more child abuse exists than was formerly thought possible. The required reporting of child abuse has brought much of the hidden abuse to the surface. Unfortunately, it is often reported long after it has happened and long after the damage has been done. Nevertheless, treatment of the abused child or adult who has been traumatized by early abuse has become the frequent subject of therapy in the offices of psychiatrists.

As with other stresses, child abuse is not always experienced by the child as "bad" or emotionally distressing. I have had a number of patients tell me that they were sexually abused in childhood by an overly friendly relative. When asked how they experienced it, some have said that for a while, they did not feel that it was "bad." Only after getting older did they realize that the adult had acted inappropriately. These individuals did not seem to be permanently scarred by the early sexual abuse.

The psychologist Erik Erikson has emphasized the need for the development of basic trust between the infant and the mothering one. If this relationship does not occur and the child cannot depend on the other person to meet his basic needs, he becomes anxious and insecure. This may have grave consequences in the child's future, as anxiety will interfere with growth in future stages of development. If the child cannot depend on and trust the mothering one, he can grow up feeling distrustful of others. At a later stage, this can evolve into a distrusting personality trait or a paranoid personality.

There is an increasing amount of research being done in the field of early childhood development. The use of videotapes of mother-child interactions, studies of twins, the effects of early childhood stimulation, and many other observations will facilitate a greater understanding of how the child develops and what can be done to foster good ego development, while minimizing stress in the early years.

Assuming that the child has had a supportive experience with his mother and/or mother substitute and hopefully a father, his next major challenge is to confront those most like him. This occurs early with siblings or when the child enters a day care program or nursery school. Children who are two to three years old usually do not play with each other as much as they play around each other. They are usually more occupied by things–objects to manipulate, such as toys. When another child takes away his toy, the child is confronted with the first challenge in asserting him or herself. Most children will do just that unless they are, by reason of temperament, not aggressive enough. Instead of expressing anger, they may cry or look for assistance from an adult. Herein lies the beginning of a series of reactions that may lead to a passive behavioral reaction to life's experiences. Other children may meet this stress with the appropriate expression of anger, followed by an adult entering the dispute to settle the matter.

Many children easily shift from one stage of life to another with relatively little apparent difficulty. Times of potential crises such as attending school for the first time, entering adolescence, going through the stages of puberty, adapting to sexual roles, and experiencing identity problems are all areas of stress. The areas of personal and sexual identity that confront adolescents will be discussed in more detail later.

ADULT STRESSES

In adult life, the choice of vocational goals and problems on the job again create considerable stress. When an individual suddenly finds herself passed over at work and not promoted, the experience can be perceived as a severe blow to her self-esteem. Another individual can lose or quit a job and yet feel very confident about finding another form of work. However, as the months wear on and she has not found a new job, self-esteem can be eroded, causing a new and unexpected stress.

In marriage, there are often stresses on relationships within the family, in the marriage partners, or with the children. As time passes, a given marriage may find husband and wife remaining relatively constant in their aspirations and feelings. However, in many marriages one or both persons may change goals and interests. Eventually, their emotional reactions to events may very considerably. Activities that were welcomed during childhood or adolescence may be viewed as frightening in adult life. Such changes can produce enormous crises in marriage. The once delicate balance can be upset, causing very disruptive phases, possibly leading to divorce. Furthermore, when the fantasies about marriage and children fall short and the reality of unmet needs becomes apparent, both partners can feel a great deal of anxiety.

Recently, a new marital stress has become more common. I am referring to marriages in which a wife earns more money than her husband. For some men, this represents a severe blow to their self-esteem, particularly when the husband has grown up in a traditional household in which the father was the sole breadwinner.

The so-called midlife crisis is not for men only. Many books have been written about this stage of life. The menopausal years, the "empty nest syndrome," and the return of children as adults to the home all have the potential for increased stress.

Men and women frequently do not find new challenges to keep them going, and they develop symptoms such as depression. With increasing age, both feel less attractive and this bothers some greatly, while others adapt to these changes easily with little stress.

Long-range goals, in terms of vocational aspirations or vaunted ambitions, are often not met. This has always presented problems for men; now, we are seeing a similar stress evolving in more women.

Maturity and retirement present very different kinds of stress, received well by some individuals and poorly by others. A retiree does poorly if he has not planned useful and interesting activities for his retirement years. The freedom to do anything at all without the constraints of time may seem like a welcome relief, but if not filled with useful and enjoyable activities, the time can become a millstone and a heavy burden.

In magazine articles we often see a list of stresses, usually ranked in order of difficulty. Although the ranking may be true for most persons, they often are not true for some. For example, the death of a spouse is usually ranked very high. This assumes that a warm, loving relationship exists in the married couple. If this is not the case, the loss may not be felt as a major stress, and the severance of the relationship would not be greatly mourned. On the other hand, a stress that for most individuals would be rated as mild could be experienced as severe for some. Taking a vacation is an example of such a stress, particularly if flying is involved.

Some of the common stresses of life are discussed here in more detail. This group of stresses by no means exhausts the list. No doubt the reader could enlarge upon them from his or her own experience in working with others.

STRESS ON THE JOB

Although the following is an example of a common vocational stress, it is also an illustration of how superficial advice would have been detrimental.

One day, a 45-year-old woman came to my office at the suggestion of her internist. The patient said that she had been under considerable tension at work, was depressed, and had developed a stomach ulcer. She asked her internist if she should change her job. Her doctor wisely answered: "I don't know. I think that it would be prudent for you to talk this over with a mental health professional."

The patient, indeed, had problems at work, but she also had marital difficulties. Furthermore, she had a tendency to hold in her feelings and somatisize her anger (that is, turn it inward). In doing this, she developed an ulcer as well as depression.

Within a six-month period of weekly psychotherapy, the patient began to feel much better. Her ulcer cleared, as verified by X ray, and she was able to identify her marital problems and work on them. As her marriage improved and she asserted herself in her interpersonal relationships, she felt much better. At that moment in time, she was given another assignment at her job, which turned out to be far more interesting.

If her internist had given her quick advice and suggested that she quit her job, she would not have learned about her faulty emotional habits, and she may have fallen into deeper trouble, perhaps losing her job and marriage. However, by examining the cause of her symptoms and working on the emotional problems, a better outcome occurred in a relatively short time.

Following the completion of psychotherapy, I did not keep in touch with this patient. But assuming that she continued to practice what she had learned in therapy, it is likely that her symptoms would not return. Thus, when these lessons are learned well, the patient can often prevent future problems from recurring.

A suggestion to the clergy: it is better not to give advice too quickly. Be careful about giving advice regarding matters in which you are not an expert. I have had patients ask me if they should buy a particular house or car, marry or not marry, divorce, stay married, or have more children. The best that we can do in these situations is listen to the thoughts that individuals have, consider the pros and cons with them, and let them make their own decisions. It is tempting to solve problems that are presented to you by giving simple answers. I have fallen into this trap on more than one occasion. It is an aspect of therapy that demands constant vigilance.

IDENTITY PROBLEMS

Some years ago the *New York Times* columnist/humorist Russell Baker wrote an article about identity. As best as I can recall, he said that in those days more and more people were asking the question, "Who am I?" He went on to say that when he was very young, he identified with one of the then-famous Hollywood cowboys, and his identity was so strong that he knew exactly who he was–Tom Mix. During adolescence, he watched Tyrone Power in the movies, and when he encountered the first girl that ever winked at him, again he had no doubt about who he was–yes, Tyrone Power.

Every few years, he had another role model until he got older, at which point he really did not want to know, "Who am I?" He was afraid of the answer! He concluded it was most important for role models to be available for identification at least until one got to the next station in life.

Although related in a humorous way, there is much truth in the need for identifying with others as we pass through various stages in life. The books *Passages* and *New Passages* by Gail Sheehy describe the stages of a woman's journey through life very well. A similar book for men is *The Seasons of a Man's Life* by Daniel J. Levinson.

Next, I would like to discuss sexual identity as well as identity roles—the way in which we become our unique selves.

Sexual Identity

Sexual identity has always been fraught with difficulty. From the early sexual explorations of childhood to the sexual trials and errors of adolescence, there are many doubts and fears that can enter a developing person's mind. Just how does sexual preference develop? It cannot be explained at all by discussing hormone levels. There seems to be no correlation between these levels and sexual preference. Rather, there is a mental/psychological inclination or preference toward the same or opposite sex. The preference for homosexual partners is reportedly between 10 to 15 percent in the general population. How do scientists account for this preference when it appears to exist almost exclusively in the human world? In the animal kingdom there is little homosexual behavior, except at times when the opposite sex is not available. What is there about humans that creates this difference? At this time, the answer is not clear. Early psychoanalytic solutions to this enigma are open to serious question. In many of the early writings of the psychoanalysts, the strong mother and the weak father were accused of setting up the scene for the production of male homosexuality. But this pattern can be seen in many marriages, and the children of such partners are much more often heterosexual. In other words, there is no consistent pattern found in the families of homosexual men.

In today's environment, in contrast to 50 years ago, the choice of sexual preference appears to be much more open than at other times. Some investigators question whether an individual has a choice at all, or whether the individual is developmentally destined toward a sexual preference. Speaking scientifically, there is no answer to this at the present time. Moralists among us believe it to be a clear choice, but in reality the problem appears to be much more complicated. I have counseled married men with children who would have preferred to stay with their families, but who felt driven to a life with a homosexual partner. They did not do this merely on impulse, but were pushed by deep mental, physical, and psychological factors that are, as yet, difficult to understand.

So, at the present level of our understanding, it is not clear how sexual identity occurs. There is little doubt that the early influence of the father and mother are important, but even their positive effect on the child will not guarantee that the sexual identity will be predictable. It remains for future investigators to solve this all-too-human mystery. Sexual identity issues are discussed further in Chapter 12, "Sexual Problems in Our Culture."

And what of the sexual revolution that has occurred? Has it led to greater satisfaction among the populace? Have there been fewer sexual problems? The answer to both questions is negative. Sexual anxiety, impotence, premature ejaculation, lack of orgasm, and other problems do not seem to have vanished with the newfound freedoms. Knowledge about STDs has lessened the prevalence of some of them, yet greater sexual freedom has facilitated the spread of other diseases. The problems in the area of sex, at best, are not less, but different.

Identity Roles

With whom did you identify as a young child, as an adolescent, or even as an adult? No doubt you identified with many individuals while growing up. Early on, the identification is either with a single parent, both parents, or a substitute parent to whom the child goes for feeding, caring, and security. Later, he is influenced by the extended family and by those involved in his education. Teachers become role models of great importance, as most of us can attest.

But, the influence of peers, which begins at about five to seven years of age, has been seriously underestimated. The child identifies with friends, takes on the characteristics of his peers, and incorporates them into his very being. At times, a child even identifies in some ways with those whom he fears. He tries on one mask after another to see which one fits best. In the end none fit; he has to be himself, a compilation of all his inherited qualities and his past sources of identity.

In the process, the loss or gain of self-esteem is an important factor in his psychological development. Some children experience severe narcissistic injury along the developmental path. Such injuries may come from overbearing, cruel, or negligent parenting or from traumatic environmental influences. Ego psychologists have emphasized the significance of these times of trauma to the developing ego. Some individuals do not progress much beyond severe injuries to their self-esteem while others, during later stages of growth, appear to overcome these psychological injuries and do well. The ability of the individual to surmount such blows to the ego seems to be dependent on his innate, inherited qualities as well as the support available from family, friends, and his environment.

Even in adult life, we are influenced by the input of our environment. Who can doubt the impact of the media, drugs, and pop culture on the general public? Our identities are affected by all of these factors and many more. A heavy burden falls on the clergy to be vigilant and point out the pernicious influences that are present in our culture and to work toward eliminating such factors. Psychotherapists and others involved in the helping professions should do their part as well.

Identity and stress are closely related. Our identity often helps us with our stress. If one is comfortable with one's identity, one feels less stress. Confusion about identity can be the source of constant stress and can lead to emotional disturbances that have physical and mental consequences.

THE STRESS OF LOSS

There is, perhaps, no greater stress one can experience than significant loss. It can involve the loss of a loved one, a job, a goal not attained, or anything that was expected but not realized. Loss can occur when possessions are taken away, illness occurs, we suffer from a loss of function, and from many other situations.

In Chapter 11, I have discussed in detail the psychology of loss, and I will not repeat it here. Suffice it to say that loss can produce great stress on the individual and result in a variety of symptoms. Even the threat of loss or the fear of losing control can cause a severe reaction.

Many years ago I saw a woman who had succeeded well in most of life's challenges until she was asked to testify in court about some financial records for which she was responsible. She had committed no crime and was not being accused of any wrongdoing. Nevertheless, having to appear in court to testify was enough to cause a severe depression that required antidepressants and psychotherapy. Her point of vulnerability–low self-esteem–became obvious. Although much improved during treatment, she had to have me ask her employer to have someone else go to court for her because she still could not cope with the anxiety of a court appearance. When she was absolved of this responsibility, her improvement was complete.

I have seen clinical depressions caused by the failure to be promoted at work, by suspected but unproven infidelity, by the rejection of close friends, and by many other real or perceived losses.

On the other hand, there are individuals who handle loss in admirable ways. Some turn misfortune into careers–the paralysis of limbs into philanthropic causes. What enables one person to do this and not another is a complex and often unpredictable phenomenon.

The clergy and psychotherapists, as well as others in the helping field, are often in the position of assisting persons who have suffered loss. Most individuals are able to overcome loss in a reasonable period of time with the support of friends, family, and the clergy. When there is continued emotional distress due to loss, psychological or psychiatric treatment may be required. The type of treatment would depend on the severity of the symptoms. For example, if the person is suffering from severe depression, it may be necessary to use antidepressant medication to facilitate the return to emotional health. In less severe cases, psychotherapy is sufficient to help the distressed individual.

MARITAL STRESS

In the process of dealing with marital problems, it has occurred to me many times that a successful marriage may be a matter of luck, good fortune, destiny, or certainly something that defies one's best intentions.

Have you had the following experience? You saw two young people marry, with all the hopes and aspirations of any marriage. Only a few short years later, they were separated and divorced. Much later, you had the opportunity to talk to one or both partners;

it was all quite understandable–how the marriage deteriorated, and what went wrong. But, could you have predicted the outcome of the marriage? I find that I cannot make such predictions with any great accuracy.

What is a good marriage? What are the ingredients that make one successful and not another? I believe that these are challenging questions, and I know no absolute answers. However, there are certain pivotal areas that I believe are important in the success or failure of any marriage. I would like to consider three such areas that often cause great stress. They are by no means all inclusive.

Incompatibility of Interests

Many marriages start too early or too impulsively, long before the couple has clearly established vocational or marriage goals. I can recall a situation in which the husband was the star athlete in high school, but a poor student. He married a classmate who admired him for his athletic prowess and popularity. After finishing high school, he went to work as a manual laborer and had no desire to further his education. This would not have been a problem if his wife felt the same way. But she had intellectual needs that were not fulfilled until she obtained further education. This caused a split in their relationship that gradually eroded the marriage. Years later, the woman in the marriage obtained a graduate degree while her husband maintained his disinterest in anything that required the use of his intellect.

There are many marriages in which one person has far more education than the other. This alone does not create incompatibility. In such a relationship, there has to be at least some interest on the part of both parties in what the other is doing–not complete disinterest. The same could be said for a marriage in which both persons are highly educated, but neither takes any interest in what the other does.

How do marriage partners maintain an appreciation of the work or interests of one another? Sometimes it comes so naturally that it appears that neither is trying at all to attend to this issue. Most often, it takes the active effort of both parties to think of and participate in the other's concerns and activities–whether or not they are successes or failures.

Is it possible for two people to be married and have very dissimilar interests? Yes, providing that there is sufficient time and areas of mutual concern that manage to occupy them. This could include the extended family, children, grandchildren, or organizations that attract them both to some degree.

If the individuals entering marriage have plenty of interests in common, they may find it easier to enjoy the marriage. This alone, however, is no guarantee of success, as there are many other important ingredients required for a successful marriage.

Sexual Incompatibility

If there is an area of great discussion in this country, it concerns the incompatibility concerning sex in marriage. Volumes have been written about it, most based on empirical data rather than research. Since I cannot contribute to the research, I will confine myself to the clinical aspects that impress me most often in my work with marriage problems. There are several areas of conflict that I have observed. They involve the frequency and quality of sexual encounters, as well as the matter of sexual rigidity.

If the desired frequency of sexual intercourse is markedly different in a married couple, it causes a great deal of stress. This occurs especially when there is impotence or frigidity present, but it is a concern even when these conditions are not present. Sexual appetites vary considerably and depend on many physical and emotional factors. Some couples live together before marriage in order to determine if they are sexually suited to each other. I have seen many cases where this was attempted, only to have things change drastically after marriage. I have had young people tell me that living together is simply "playing house." It is very different from marriage, where commitment and responsibility play an important role.

In some marriages there are very big differences between the two partners; one has little or no need for sex while the other has a regularly felt need for a sexual outlet. In our culture it is usually the husband who complains of inadequate sexual experiences while his wife complains of her husband's preoccupation with sex. In such instances, the woman's complaint is that her emotional needs for attention, affection, and caressing–without sex–are not being met. Such complaints are often followed by the wife's threat that if her emotional needs are not realized, then the sexual needs of the husband will not be met either. Such a standoff may be enough for some couples to consider divorce.

The quality of the sexual experience is hard to measure and depends on many factors. It is, perhaps, more related to the degree that the marriage partners can communicate with each other than anything else. The need for effective communication in general is necessary even before any sexual encounter occurs. If a poor relationship exists and communication is at a low ebb, one would hardly expect the sexual act to be very satisfactory. But even during the sexual experience itself, communication via the various senses must occur to a certain degree in order for the quality of the sex act to be satisfactory.

The quality of sexual encounters is also dependent on the lack of rigidity on the part of the couple. If one has a compulsive way of doing things and cannot experiment with various methods and positions, the experience may not be very satisfying. With education and marital counseling, such problems of rigidity can often be altered. If both parties are rigid and compulsive, there may be no problem.

Marital therapy can often be of considerable help in assisting the stress that occurs in a marriage with sexual difficulties. In my experience the Masters and Johnson techniques have been most helpful. They stress sensate focusing as a method to assist those who have problems of rigidity, a lack of sexual desire, and difficulties with orgasm. The technique basically is a way of concentrating on the physical needs of the other person in order to arouse the most pleasant sensual feelings in all areas of the body, sexual and non-sexual. This treatment method assumes that emotionally the couple are congruent and really want to improve their sexual relationship (Kaplan, 1974, pp. 208-214). For further detail on this type of treatment, the reader should consult the works of Masters and Johnson.

There are many more problems concerning sex and marriage that could fill volumes. The clergyperson can attempt to address any sexual problems that a congregant feels free to discuss, but his usefulness may depend on his experience and training in this area. And if a clergyperson feels he is being asked about a marriage problem with which he feels uncomfortable, he should recommend that a trained psychotherapist be consulted. Some congregants may resist seeing someone else because of embarrassment due to the sexual nature of the problem. It is important that the clergyperson make it clear to the couple that he does not feel expert in this area. Furthermore, it should be pointed out that the initial hesitation to seek the advice of another will be quickly overcome after the first few sessions with the other therapist, assuming that the latter is compatible with the couple. For more on the subject of psychotherapists and how to chose them, see Chapter 16, "Psychotherapists: Who, What, Why, and When to Refer."

Philosophical Differences in Marriage

When I was growing up, one of the marriage problems that I heard about frequently concerned the differences a couple had as the result of their religious beliefs. In my background, the issues were usually Catholic versus Protestant or strong religious beliefs versus no particular interest in any faith. Many a serious marital battle was waged around these closely held views. Today, it is less likely that this is the case in our society except among Fundamentalist groups of any faith, where definitive religious beliefs are of great concern in marriage. Similar concerns also exist between families of Catholic and Jewish faith.

As time has gone on, there has been less attention paid to religious differences by the general public. Intermarriage between faiths has become increasingly common. I have seen problems in such marriages, but not necessarily because of religious differences. The religious concerns appear to have been diluted somewhat in the more accepting view that society has developed. One could speculate as to why this has happened. Nevertheless, in some families, religious differences cause bitter feelings and can lead to difficult marriage problems.

While religious diversity in marriage seems to be on the decline as a problem in the minds of the general public, other issues have attained more importance. I refer especially to women's roles in our society and women's rights. There have been many victories for women, but many heartaches as well. In vocational pursuits, professions, industry, and the military, women are now occupying jobs formerly held by men. And their new freedoms have extended into many other areas. But in marriage the changes have also produced some problems. There are men who have not been able to tolerate the role change that women have desired. Some women are not entirely certain that the new freedom has been to their advantage. It seems to me that the changes have eliminated some problems and produced others. The role of women has been altered significantly; there will be no turning back, and, no doubt, more changes are yet to come. The institution of marriage will have to change along with the roles that women assume.

I have seen more than one marriage break up because of the failure of husbands to accept the role changes in their wives. On the other hand, I have witnessed rather remarkable adjustments in marriages that were originally rather traditional. The end of the twentieth century is bringing about rapid alterations in our society, making it more and more difficult for marriages to be secure and stable. It is hard to imagine what married life will be like in the twenty-first century. There is little doubt that it will be remarkably different.

COPING WITH STRESS

I am impressed with how little the average person knows about dealing with stress. Rather, most individuals simply want to know what medicine they can take to alleviate stress quickly. Our culture emphasizes orality. If you feel pain of any kind, take something for it. From pain pills to tranquilizers, this country surpasses all others in its devotion to medication for the relief of discomfort. Has anyone forgotten the commercial, "How do you spell relief? R-o-l-a-i-d-s"? But many other options are open to anyone who is willing to look within herself and think about her needs. Doing so will open up the door to dealing successfully with many stresses. The relief of stress is not accomplished best by taking drugs, alcohol, or pills. It may be much more effectively handled by considering one's internal resources. The process may take longer, but it will be more beneficial.

EXPLORING NEEDS

It is surprising how many educated people do not understand their needs. To put it plainly, they do not know what's good for them. Beyond that, if it is made clear what their needs are, there is a tremendous resistance to obtaining what would no doubt make them feel considerably better.

One of my patients complained about chest pains that were known to be of no medical significance. She thought she had heart disease, but after many examinations, no physician was able to uncover any sign of cardiac problems. She was advised to take regular walks but failed to do so because she claimed the weather was too cold. As the climate improved, I asked her if she had taken any walks, and she invariably replied, "I will when the weather improves." On one really gorgeous spring day I asked, "Did you walk today?" Without really thinking about it she replied, "No, but I will when the weather gets a little better." Clearly, this patient was never going to take the simple advice to exercise. Let us examine some basic needs that all humans possess to one degree or another.

Physical Needs

In recent years there has been more emphasis on physical conditioning. After being overly dependent on the automobile for too long, many people have realized that exercise may be important to health. Physicians have been late in reaching this realization and have not set the best example until a few years ago. Now individuals of all ages are walking, running, or engaging in sports as never before.

Physical conditioning has been stressed because it can prevent certain ailments, keep down weight gain, and improve the general feeling of well-being. We all know people in their thirties or forties who look like they are 10 to 15 years older because of lack of self-care and the failure to exercise. Those who exercise regularly will attest to the fact that they feel more energetic and fit, which, incidently, has an effect on self-esteem. So, why doesn't everyone exercise? The excuses go on and on: "I have no time. I can't get myself to do it. I don't have the discipline to keep at it." Some might even call it laziness. Whatever it is, the initial hurdle of resistance must be overcome before one can reap the benefits of regular exercise.

Emotional Needs

We all have the necessity to express ourselves by various means emotionally. It is important to laugh, to cry, to become angry, to caress, to love, and to experience the wide array of emotions with which humans are endowed. The basic problem in expressing human emotions is that all too often we become angry at the wrong times; we laugh at ill-chosen moments or we fail to cry when it would be appropriate to the situation. In other words, whatever the emotion felt, it is expressed inappropriately in relationship to the events happening at any given time. For example, if someone makes you angry, it might be much more appropriate to tell the other person, "What you just said makes me angry!" than to yell and scream at him. It is the appropriateness of the emotional response that determines whether the interaction will be handled in a healthy manner. At other times it might be most appropriate to yell and scream. It depends on the circumstance and to some extent on the temperament of the individual.

But what about those among us who have, by nature, never expressed themselves emotionally to the same degree as the average individual? Such persons may do well with their low-key reactions to things. They may have no inherent need to express themselves effusively. Or, they may suffer from symptoms related to their lack of emotional response to events in their lives.

When one reacts excessively to emotional situations or fails to react sufficiently, it is most important to be aware of such responses since excessive stress may develop when one does not deal well with emotions. It is often necessary to obtain professional help to handle such problems. At the same time spiritual help can be very beneficial in reframing one's outlook in emotional areas since a person's vantage point often determines whether she sees a situation as stressful.

Intellectual Needs

How many times have you seen congregants who are well-educated and do very little to feed their intellectual needs? On the other hand, how often have you witnessed the opening of the mind of the uneducated by attention to intellectual needs. I have seen those with little formal education who have read extensively and are well informed. There are also many who have obtained an education for the purposes of getting a job and then have abandoned any further intellectual pursuits.

For those who have intellectual needs and have ignored them, this is an important area to consider. Perhaps a good book or a course at a community college or vocational/technical school is appropriate to begin the process. It is important to recognize needs that are present in order to avoid emotional disturbances and subsequent symptoms. This goes for intellectual needs as well as other needs.

Creative Needs

There are individuals who have been creative since they were children. Creativity seems to ooze out of them with little effort. Such persons have no trouble keeping in touch with their creative side. But what about the rest of us? Do we also have a creative side? I believe that most of us do have some creativity, but we do not try to relate to it. Perhaps a talent for designing with color or drawing, painting, or music. But, how long have these creative talents been dormant? "I don't have the time. I'm really not that good at it." Such are the excuses. But one's life can be enriched greatly by attending to even minor creative abilities. The trick is to get started and not allow self-doubt and self-criticism to enter the picture. Some individuals have difficulty expressing their creativity because they feel that they must be experts in whatever they do, including their creative choices. Some compromise in perfectionistic ideals may be necessary for the person to enjoy modest success in expressing creative needs.

Spiritual Needs

I venture to say that even some very religious persons are not very attuned to their spiritual needs. Some practice religion as if it were a compulsion, which, if not played out in a ritualistic fashion, causes anxiety. Such religiosity contains little spirituality.

Rather, I am talking about being attuned to the needs of others; to being attentive to family, friends, and the world at large; and to meeting the needs of others and thereby meeting our own spiritual needs. A deep feeling of spiritual relationship to God, without a positive relationship to our fellow man, defeats the human benefit of religion and denies a true attentiveness to spiritual needs. As part of attending to spiritual needs, I feel that many persons neglect the emotional healing that can be the result of prayer. In the words of Tennyson in the *Idylls of the King*:

More things are wrought by prayer
Than this world dreams of—
For what are men better than sheep and goats
That nourish a blind life within the brain,
If, knowing God, they lift not hands of prayer
Both for themselves and those who call them friend?
For so the whole round earth is every way
Bound by gold chains about the feet of God.

It is the clergy, of course, who can best make their congregants aware of their spiritual needs. In the modern secular world there is little attention given to the spiritual needs of the individual. Our religious institutions and the clergy are struggling to adequately meet these needs, but spiritual needs are present in all of us. It is up to the individual, with the help of the clergy, to look into himself in order to get in touch with his spiritual side and meet these needs.

It is surprising to me that so many people have no idea about basic needs. The clergy can help their congregants become aware of such needs, and be an emotional catalyst in getting congregants started toward meeting these needs.

Psychotherapists regularly focus their client's attention to emotional needs, sometimes to the neglect of other realities that may be equally important. We are all physical, intellectual, emotional, creative, and spiritual beings—even if we neglect one or the other of these basic needs.

In addition to the suggestions given here, I have found it helpful for some patients to use meditation and relaxation techniques to deal with stress. There are many books now available in the popular press on meditation as well as relaxation training (Benson) and creative imagery (Gawain). Some may find the use of audiotapes very helpful for relaxation (Griswald). These are relaxation tapes with short messages on a variety of subjects such as sleep, concentration, losing weight, improving memory, etc. Another tape by Melzack and Perry is very helpful for the relief of chronic pain through relaxation.

Whatever medium one may use, these auxiliary methods are very helpful, but each person has to pick and chose until he finds one that suits him best. There is no one method that is totally helpful for everyone.

Only by paying attention to and meeting our basic needs can we expect to live a fulfilling life as free from harmful stress as possible. The trick is not to avoid all stress; that is not living. While being aware of our limits for stressors, we should embrace the stress that we can endure so as to live as productively and joyously as possible.

Chapter 15

Pastoral Ethics: A Psychiatrist's View

It may appear presumptuous for a psychiatrist to write about ethics when addressing readers who are predominantly clergypersons or clergy. However, in light of the all-too-frequent ethical problems of the clergy that have been receiving national attention in the media recently, it does not seem out of order to raise the topic for discussion.

Clergypersons appear to be subject to the same frailties as others, despite the high expectations of those who attend religious institutions. Even the general public is surprised when clergy are involved in ethical problems. More is expected of the clergy than of the average citizen. By the nature of his or her profession, the clergyperson is presumed to be dedicated to live an exemplary life. Perhaps these are not unreasonable expectations, but even the most sophisticated among us is somewhat surprised when a clergyperson falls from grace and exhibits very human foibles.

The clergy, like others who are in close contact with clients, can become easily enmeshed in the emotional lives of needy individuals. It is the clergy that are often on the front line. They are frequently the first to become involved with the needs of their congregants, often before the physician or the psychotherapist. It is at such times of heightened emotions and exaggerated stress that the clergy should be most alert to ethical issues. Consideration of such ethical concerns prior to the occurrence of problems may save the clergyperson considerable pain and embarrassment in his or her work.

At least four aspects involving ethics are likely to arise in the life of any active clergyperson. They will be considered under the following headings: confidentiality, transference, countertransference, and commitment.

219

CONFIDENTIALITY

How much of what a congregant tells you should be confidential? Can you talk with friends or family without violating your congregant's confidentiality? Should you give advice about a member to persons who know him or her? How "confidential" can you be with adolescents? What do you do with information that implies danger to the person's self or others? Such questions and many others may be familiar to the experienced therapist, but may be new or unusual to the beginner, be that person clergy or another professional.

Confidentiality is based on trust. Many individuals have been terribly traumatized early in life by the failure of caregivers to provide some basic trust in the formative years. If a young infant cannot depend on being fed, bathed, and clothed with some regularity, an attitude of fear and apprehension develops. Later, as the personality develops, this may be conceptualized as doubt, suspicion, and even paranoia.

In the role of counselor, the clergyperson or psychotherapist can be faced with a long therapeutic challenge in an attempt to restore even minimal trust in a person who has been deprived of the basic mutual trusting confidence that good childrearing should provide.

Some individuals insist upon an excessive amount of trust and confidentiality while others readily tell the whole world about their counseling with a therapist. However, the particular attitude of the client should not influence the counselor's basic way of dealing with the issue of confidentiality. I know of no law that states that a clergyperson must hold in confidence everything revealed by a congregant. There is such a law for physicians, depending somewhat on the state or country in which the physician practices. However, I think it is safe to say that most clergypersons feel that when they counsel members, a measure of confidentiality is implied; counseling without confidentiality would soon end.

The first rule of confidentiality is that nothing that the person reveals in a session should be told to anyone without the express consent of the counseled person. There is one exception to this rule. When the person in counseling reveals that he is about to do something dangerous to himself or others, such important information must be told to the responsible individuals involved, usually family members. This is a basic ethical tenet that psychiatrists and most other counselors follow. In practice, most clients will not object to the gathering of information from a spouse or other relatives, and most counselors see the necessity for requesting assistance from outside sources if it is clear that the client is in deep psychological trouble.

For example, if a person stated that he was planning suicide or was about to do something violent, the therapist should feel the necessity to inform relatives and/or police officials. I know of no psychotherapist or counselor who would not follow this rule. However, there is one exception to this generalization. I recently received a call from a Roman Catholic priest who had talked to a woman in confession. She stated that she was planning to kill someone. He asked me what he should do. I told him what I would do, namely, inform the police and the person whose life was in danger. He, however, told me that he was under the constraints of the confessional, and that his vows forbid him from revealing anything to anyone. Given this rule, with which the priest had to live, he had no alternative but to counsel his parishioner to refrain from killing and seek alternative help. I know of no other situation in which such a principle applies. Recent legal cases clearly indicate that psychotherapists must inform the police and the person threatened. Failure to do so makes the counselor liable to a malpractice suit.

Talking with the Family

In general, relatives do not want to know details about what is discussed in the counseling sessions; a spouse or parent usually wants to know if the therapeutic work is proceeding in a positive direction. Also, most relatives want to know if they can be helpful and will ask specifically what they can do. However, some persistent relatives can create problems. For example, let us assume that you have a husband's permission to speak with his wife, and you have knowledge of his relationship with another woman. It goes without saying that you are not free to discuss this information with the spouse. But suppose she asks you directly, "Is my husband having an affair?" You cannot answer this directly, and indirect answers could be too revealing. If you were to say, "Confidentiality does not permit me to discuss certain information," this would imply that there may be things that are hidden.

A more confronting way of answering this question is to say, "Why are you asking me?" This may give the impression of avoiding the question. Perhaps that best way to address the spouse's question is, "I think you should ask your husband that question, since it concerns important matters between you," or, "Your question implies that you are doubting your husband's loyalty and commitment to you. These things should be talked about together between husband and wife."

Sometimes individuals who are upset may consciously or unconsciously trap a counselor by demanding confidentiality about information that really should not remain private. Adolescents often put it this way, "I want to tell you something, but I want you to promise not to tell anyone about it." Some counselors, especially neophytes who are eager to ingratiate the person, may fall into this trap and agree to keep the information confidential. Following such a concession by the therapist or counselor, the adolescent may speak of dire things such as his intention to take his life or some other violent act.

How should one react to an attempt on the part of the counselee to extract such promises? I generally agree with my patients that I should hold things in confidence, but I inform them of conditions where this is not possible, namely, when I perceive that the information that I am hearing is of definite harm to the patients or to someone else. This usually refers to physical harm, such as suicide and homicide. If a person threatened to do harm to himself or others, I would enquire at great length as to the purpose and motive of the threat. If such a threat appeared to be serious, I would have to consider the use of antidepressant medication or possibly hospitalization. If a clergyperson was the first person to hear such a threat, it would be prudent for him to refer the congregant to a psychotherapist for further evaluation. In addition, the person's family should be informed of the serious nature of the problem.

Although areas of confidentiality should be preserved, I feel it is important that the clergyperson maintain contact with the family of adolescents because the latter are subject to such lability of mood and emotional reactions. A good working relationship with parents and teenagers is possible if the ground rules are established early in the counseling. Generally, it should be borne in mind that, as noted, parents are not as concerned about details as they are about the direction of their child's life and the ways in which they can help their youngsters. I recall my own concern when my son, who was then in junior high school, told me that he was attending group sessions in school with a social worker. I wanted to know why this was happening. The counselor informed me that the group was formed to talk about typical problems encountered in the teenage years. After assuring me that there was no crisis or unusual concerns about my son, I felt relieved. The details of what was discussed were of no great interest to me.

I have had long-term patients tell me that it took many sessions, and in some cases, years to finally trust me enough to reveal some of their feelings about significant figures in their lives. For many patients, it is even more difficult to express feelings and emotions that are occurring in the session itself, especially feelings about the therapy or the therapist. When such emotions are expressed by the patient, it may be very important; what occurs in the therapeutic hour may simulate the repeated daily interactions of patients in their lives outside the consulting room. More about this follows.

TRANSFERENCE AND COUNTERTRANSFERENCE PROBLEMS

In order to deal with the previously explained interactions, it is important to first understand the origin of these concepts. We commonly observe in ourselves and others the tendency to behave in similar ways from day to day. With certain exceptions, a person's general decorum will not differ much from week to week. Over the years, some individuals do change. Such things as severe trauma, dramatic emotional events, and religious conversions can cause remarkable changes, but they are exceptions.

Freud first observed this phenomenon while engaged in his psychoanalytic work. He noted that people repeated patterns in their lives with remarkable frequency. He called this tendency the repetition compulsion. That is, the behavior of individuals does not differ much from year to year or from one situation to another.

In therapy, such repetitions can be observed in the reaction of the client to his counselor, the patient to her therapist. It is common in the course of psychotherapy to have a patient react to the therapist as though he were a person from the patient's past. Such a condition occurs when a patient unconsciously takes feelings and attitudes from the past and applies them to the present in the therapeutic situation. For example, if a patient had a severe, dominating father, he might be very sensitive to the minor perceived criticisms of the therapist, even if the latter was trying to be very delicate with the use of constructive comments. Or, if a female patient never felt secure that she had the full concern and affection of her father, she might attempt to please the therapist in a number of ways, some of which might be overtly seductive. Freud called this process transference.

It is in the area of transference that therapists and clergy often confront ethical problems. Transference may be set off by such qualities in the counselor as a kind, empathic manner; a controlling, confident, in-charge nature; or any other qualities that are reminiscent of the patient's emotional background. The reaction depends on the past psychology of the person requiring the counseling. If the counselor is a clergyperson, and he reacts to such a transference situation as though it were a normal social interaction, he could quickly become emotionally involved with the congregant. The failure to recognize this interaction as a transference relationship could cause serious damage to the clergyperson's role, including his effectiveness as a counselor. The following example will illustrate how a transference occurs and how it can be handled.

A 35-year-old married woman began psychotherapy with me for symptoms of depression and anxiety. A positive relationship was soon established. However, she appeared inordinately interested in my personal life and asked frequent questions about my outside activities. Patients may do this on occasion out of friendliness and a need to socialize the professional situation. But this patient appeared to enjoy my attention, and made it obvious that coming to therapy was a high point in her life.

After several months of therapy, the patient began to speak of my kindness, gentleness, and empathic manner. These qualities were certainly exaggerated, as on other occasions, I have had patients refer to me as cold and withdrawn. As with judging art, what one observes as pleasing is based on the eye of the beholder.

Soon the patient admitted to very positive feelings and stated that she was in love with me. Such inappropriate emotions can occur in psychotherapy or any form of counseling and have been the subject of intense drama in the theater, movies, and television. But such positive transference represents a serious part of therapy, and it must be dealt with sensitively.

In this particular case, the patient had an unresolved relationship with her alcoholic father, who was often sullen and angry. At times her father was understanding and gentle, but this was all too infrequent. When she encountered these traits in me, her therapist, she felt a closeness and bonding that was out of proportion to the reality of the situation. These feelings became intense, and the patient expressed this as romantic love. At such times, it is very important for the therapist to understand the historical roots of these emotions. The transference nature of the reaction has to be made clear to the patient. The therapist can acknowledge the feelings that the patient has for him without personalizing and socializing the relationship.

As time went on, my patient gradually began to learn how the present therapeutic situation was a repetition of the past relationship with her father. Furthermore, she became aware of her tendency to fall in love with teachers, employers, or others in authority–those who showed interest in her. Several of these involvements caused considerable emotional pain for her in the past.

The resolution of transference phenomenon can be very therapeutic. Much emotional distress can be avoided by understanding the nature of transference. When understood in the context of psychotherapy, it has been referred to by therapists as a corrective emotional experience.

There is another form of transference that is important for the clergy. It is called projective identification.

I recall a patient, named John, who made me feel inadequate and ineffective. He asked frequent questions about the treatment of his depression and the use of medications. These were not unusual questions, but he also asked me about financial matters and whether to buy a smaller home or a new car. I explored the questions to find out what basically concerned him. I had no intention of telling him what to buy or advising him on financial matters. He pressed me to give answers. When I refused, he implied that I was not helpful; he complained that I did not talk enough, and questioned my concern for his welfare. My perception of him was that he suffered from marked ambivalence about making decisions and wanted me to decide things for him as his father had done in the past. Because of the persistent nature of his complaints, I felt annoyed and truly ineffective.

In the process of projective identification, the person ascribes to the therapist negative qualities that he or she feels. In this example, John projected onto me his own ambivalence and anxiety, as though it was I who could not make decisions. Then, by consistently maintaining this stance, he pressured me into feeling discontent with my role as a psychotherapist. Thus, without being consciously aware of it, he interfered with my goal of allowing him to make deliberate and conscious decisions for himself. In his personal relationships with others, John behaved much the same way. He made his friends and family feel that they were not helpful and even useless to him.

Let me present another illustration. When a person feels impotent and powerless, he or she can project onto the therapist or clergyperson an image of omnipotence. This can be as distressing to the helper as the projection of inadequacies can foster discontent with one's caregiving abilities; it does not take long for the omnipotent one to fall or to reveal feet of clay, resulting in further disappointment on the part of the person seeking help.

As a clergyperson, you should be aware that certain individuals are capable of making you feel pressured and inadequate even when you are doing a competent job. Or, when a congregant aggrandizes you or is excessively critical, it may be the result of the mechanism of projective identification.

COUNTERTRANSFERENCE

Freud recognized that the therapist could also have transference experiences while engaged in the very work of doing psychotherapy. Freud called this countertransference. It occurs when the therapist has an exaggerated reaction to the patient based on the therapist's past experiences with significant persons in his own background. Thus, certain personality traits or physical and emotional reactions of the patient may trigger feelings in the therapist that at first may be very hard to understand. The reason for the reaction is unconscious; it may be positive or negative in nature. The therapist may feel unduly attached to or upset with the patient. Often, these emotions can be resolved. At times it may require considerable personal analysis on the part of the therapist to reach back into his own past in order to identify the source of the unusual feelings toward the patient.

Because of the heightened emotional charge involved in the relationship between therapist and client, both the counselor and the counseled can become involved in ethical problems that are unique to the consulting room. If the therapist has unexplained emotional reactions of anger, love, or other unusual feelings, he can understand such feelings if they are examined in the light of his own past emotional life. The following example will illustrate how this happens.

One day, a colleague approached me and told me that he was very upset with one of his patients. The patient was somewhat older than my friend and had a very overbearing manner. At times the patient could be very confronting and angry, qualities that normally would not bother this therapist. He usually could deal with such traits quite appropriately.

It took some soul-searching for the therapist to appreciate the countertransference aspects of the situation. Upon reflection, the therapist realized that he was responding to some unresolved conflicts in his past, which the patient had elicited. He recognized that the irrational anger that his patient at times displayed was similar to what he experienced with his father in the past.

When the anxiety first developed, the therapist had no idea of its origin; he was quite alarmed and puzzled by these uncomfortable feelings. When he became aware of the countertransference aspects of the therapy, he was gradually able to overcome his anxiety.

It was Freud's opinion that a positive transference was necessary to bring about a therapeutic relationship with a patient. In practice, both positive and negative transference are regarded as very important ingredients of therapy. A counselor must know when a person's reactions are based on the usual and expected emotional reactions or whether they represent transference phenomena. Failure to do so can result in serious ethical problems and emotional distress on the part of the counselor. In a similar manner, the therapist or clergyperson should recognize his or her unusual reactions to others. Such phenomena may be the result of past experiences rather than be simply based on the here and now; they may be countertransference issues.

COMMITMENT

How much time should you give to a congregant? How do you know when you are "burned out"? Should your needs ever come first? Is there a time to ask for help? How do you fit your family needs into your busy schedule? Do you ever place your family before your work responsibilities? How much devotion to your job is enough? Do you know when to stop? There are questions that have to be addressed at various stages of one's career. Failure to do so can result in emotional and ethical dilemmas.

The Counselor's Basic Needs

It is interesting to ask individuals why they elected to enter the particular field in which they work. People in the helping professions, such as teachers, nurses, physicians, clergymen, and mental health professionals all have their own reasons for entering their particular field. Upon close inquiry, one usually uncovers a need to help, which is born out of early experiences that are either traumatic or especially meaningful because of highly significant and emotionally inspiring persons in one's past.

For example, many teachers have been influenced positively by their past teachers who were good role models. Others have had very negative experiences with their childhood instructors, and they consciously or unconsciously want to correct these bad memories by being good examples in their own lives. Nurses, physicians, and mental health workers often recall poor parenting or a traumatic childhood, which led them to choose their particular profession. A nurse may be very sensitive to the needs of long-term patients because of a family member that suffered from a chronic illness. Persons who grow up in homes with alcoholism frequently become mental health workers. And, of course, those who enter the clergy are motivated by similar forces from their past. In our own lives, we often try to provide for others the emotional support that we felt was deficient in our past.

Time for Self

I have seen individuals in the helping professions who simply worked too hard. Whether it was caused by devotion to the job, an obsessive need to work, or whatever reason, it was plain to everyone that the job had become too time-consuming in the person's life. I recall a physician in private practice who never seemed to finish her chart work. Papers were piled high on her desk. She worked far into the night to complete them, but it never seemed to result in a smaller pile. Instead of refusing to accept new patients, she accepted more and more. Finally, she had to quit her practice and move on to another form of work that did not require her obsessive attention. Although still very conscientious, she was able to handle the new job and be very successful at it.

Sometimes this need to work excessively is based on a low self-esteem, an inordinate need to be wanted, a compulsive need to do well, or a misdirected and overactive superego. Whatever the reason for overworking, it is clear that it is not in the best interest of the worker to do so. One has to conclude that the priorities with which the person is working are out of order. Such individuals often have the mistaken belief that the needs of others are always more important than the person's own needs.

I have heard patients express the idea that to be concerned about one's own needs is selfish, and that the needs of others should always come first. I can recall being caught in this kind of bind, in which I was functioning in a compulsive way, giving in to the needs of others while neglecting my own. In my fourth year of medical school, through sheer fatigue and excessive work, this caused a three-week illness with high fever and pneumonia.

On a simpler level, I can remember sitting at dinner with a group of fellow interns. I was called by phone and told that there was a patient waiting for me in the clinic. It was not an emergency, but I left my half-eaten dinner and went off to see the patient. Before leaving, I told the others where I was going. They asked why I did not finish eating dinner, which would have taken only a few more minutes. At the time, I felt that they were being very callous, and that it just was not right for me to keep a patient waiting. Since then, I have learned that it is more important to take care of one's own needs, and that with the exception of emergencies, one works best when basic needs are met.

Perhaps a better example is the adjustment that I had to make in my daily schedule when I began my private practice. At that time, I had the good fortune of having many more referrals than I could handle. It was difficult to refuse patients, particularly when they were referred by doctors whom I knew well. I could manage a certain number of patients in a given week, but when the numbers increased by two or three beyond my usual number, I became irritable and depressed. I then knew to back off, and refuse to take on more patients for the sake of my own mental health and the welfare of my patients and my family.

To know intellectually that one should not overwork may not be enough to prevent a counselor from doing so. A compulsive nature, a driving ambition, a need to overcompensate for feelings of inferiority–all of these factors may interfere with sound judgment in this matter. But failure to take care of one's own physical and emotional needs will inevitably result in distressing symptoms and poor performance.

I have often talked to the wives of busy executives, doctors, and others who have complained bitterly about the lack of time that they have been able to spend with their husbands. The husbands were very successful in their work and tended to be compulsively driven in their jobs. Often there was pride in the comment, "I haven't taken a vacation in five years." In some distorted way, this was worn as a badge to the world that the individual was an unusual being who deserved special credit for his masochistic obedience to conscience. Meanwhile, the successful executive or physician left behind unresolved problems in his family.

Other Needs

It may appear to be elementary that we all have basic needs. The need to work is very basic, but like every need it can be grossly overdone. Other needs are equally important but are overlooked by the busy worker. The need to express a variety of emotions such as anger, laughter, sorrow, hurt, joy, optimism, and many other human feelings has been documented in the work of therapists for years. When emotions are thwarted, symptoms can ensue. These may be seen in the emotional or in the physical area. Anxiety, depression, panic, and psychosomatic illnesses are very common. When anger is not expressed appropriately, it is often felt as depression or anxiety. Therapists are by no means immune to the same stress and emotions experienced by their clients.

If the counselor begins to feel excessive anxiety or any other symptom that interferes with her ability to function, she should first do an inventory of her life to ascertain whether her needs are being met. If priorities can be assessed and changes can be made, symptoms may disappear. However, if in spite of efforts toward self-correction, symptoms still persist, the counselor would do well to seek outside assistance toward solving her emotional problems.

I have treated members of the clergy and their families and found them to have the same problems that others have. Neglect of children, indifference to the needs of family members, sexual indiscretions, and failure to attend to emotional and physical needs are all too common in the lives of active clergypersons.

Perhaps the most outstanding trait present in this group is the desire to solve all problems alone. Frequently I have heard religious people, including the clergy, say that they did not believe in the psychological approach to emotional problems. They attempted to work it all out in a religious way, through prayer and devotions. I know of one clergyperson who did this for a period of two years, even though she was suicidal for a good part of this time. Psychiatric help with the use of medication would have shortened the illness to perhaps a few months.

The excessive giving of the self to others can sometimes lead to what is commonly called burnout. It can occur when the clergyperson is overworked, does not attend to her needs, or the individual has been at the job too long. It may also occur when the religious leader loses her grasp on her faith, or when her work becomes too routine.

Burnout happens when the emotional life of the counselor does not progress evenly with the work. Many years ago, I spoke with a missionary who had spent 20 years in China. He said that the hardest part of his job was the constant giving to his parishioners without being able to receive spiritual nourishment from any outside source. When he was able to go home to the United States or attend a conference with other workers in China, he was refreshed and able to continue his work. It seems clear that periodic physical, emotional, and spiritual refueling is necessary to keep one's energy level high.

Another aspect of burnout is the lack of internal stimuli leading to boredom. One way to look at boredom is to consider it the result of routine, of constant repetition. Perhaps this is so. For me, it is more helpful to put it in terms of the person not doing something that he could be doing. That is, when bored, one can ask the question, "What is it that I could be doing that I am not doing in the present situation?" Answering this question can often lead to a solution to the experienced boredom.

Some counselors have the illusion that they can do everything by themselves. Psychotherapists refer to this as rescue fantasies. The individual feels that only he can do the job. This person is of the opinion that no one else could possibly understand the person as well as he can. Where others have failed, this person will prevail and will rescue the individual from his distress. Such counselors are particularly apt to fall into the transference problems referred to earlier in this chapter.

Commitment to work is a noble ethical concern. When commitment exceeds the ability of an individual's capacity, it is no longer virtuous. The clergyperson should be responsible for his own life, meet his commitments, but also give due regard to his own emotional and physical needs.

SUMMARY

The areas of confidentiality, transference, countertransference, and commitment can lead to much distress for the active clergyperson. Emotional upheavals resulting in personal stress and consequent stress on one's family are very common. Often these situations can be resolved by reflection on the work being done. It is important to be observant and somewhat analytical in regard to these matters.

Perhaps the most dangerous approach is to try to always handle everything alone. Failing to recognize the need for the advice of colleagues, who may be more objective, may represent a fatal flaw in the clergyperson's personality. If after consulting with a trusted friend or colleague, the issue is still not clear, it would be very appropriate for the clergyperson to seek the advice of a trained counselor. This need not be a psychiatrist, but the individual should be skilled in analyzing the previously mentioned problems. Failure to do so could cause an ethical dilemma and needless suffering.

Chapter 16

Psychotherapists: Who, What, Why, and When To Refer

The famous American psychologist William James once wrote the following insightful comment: "If you believe well of your fellow men, you may create the good you believe in." This can be applied to the process of psychotherapy when the therapy is being conducted by a competent and well-trained therapist. It is important that the therapist is able to recognize the healthy areas of the patient's mind as well as the pathological areas. In the intact part of the patient's mental functioning, the therapist should be able to see the potential for growth, while in the sick part of the mind, he or she should recognize the possibilities for healing.

However, a neophyte or poorly trained psychotherapist can be deluded into thinking that the patient's pathology will always respond to the therapists' believing creativity, that is, new therapists sometimes believe that if they try hard enough or are creative enough, they can cure any psychological illness. Confidence in one's ability is necessary, but not sufficient in itself to do good therapy. I have known therapists in various fields who were clearly trying to work with patients who had pathology for which the therapist was poorly trained. In order to do the best possible psychotherapy, there is no substitute for thorough training at a recognized institution.

There are psychotherapists who are trained pastoral counselors, social workers, psychologists, drug and alcohol counselors, vocational and rehabilitation counselors, and other types of counselors. Besides the variety of therapists, all psychiatrists are not psychotherapists, just as all social workers and psychologists are not psychotherapists. They can be involved in a variety of occupations such as research; academic, forensic or administrative pursuits; and other activities.

To the emotionally distraught individual, this must be very confusing. How, then, can a person choose a psychotherapist? With whom can one feel free to reveal highly confidential material? Who can one trust? And how can you as a clergyperson be helpful in assisting your congregant in obtaining competent psychotherapy when needed?

THE PSYCHIATRIST'S EDUCATION

Since I am not expert in all the specific qualifications of the mentioned therapists, I will elaborate only on the background and training of psychiatrists.

After graduation from a recognized four-year college, completing a full medical school curriculum and acquiring a medical degree, it is required that the graduate enter a residency program for four years of further training in the general area of psychiatry.

At first, the resident physician is expected to have considerable experience in the care of hospitalized patients for the treatment of the more severe psychotic disorders such as schizophrenic disorder, bipolar disorder (manic-depressive disorder), organic mental disorders, as well as neurological and psychosomatic problems. Many hours of outpatient work with patients who have neurotic and personality disorders also are required. These patients are usually seen on a weekly or semi-weekly basis for psychotherapy, while under the careful supervision of senior psychiatrists.

Other subjects in the training include substance abuse, the use of psychotropic medications, child and adolescent psychiatry, and family, group, and individual therapy. Consideration is given to psychotherapy of all kinds—dynamic (analytic) psychotherapy, supportive, behavioral, cognitive, and short-term therapy.

In most programs, various theories of psychological development are explored. Although there may be greater emphasis on one authority than on another, most training is eclectic in nature; that is, not strictly Freudian, Adlerian, or Jungian in theory. There is no authority exclusively taught, but rather the best of various theories are used. Whatever is applicable and useful for a given patient is applied in therapy.

Most training centers have the view, which I share, that a therapist who follows one authority alone and does not entertain other options is compromising his or her therapeutic ability by having such a narrow focus. For example, some patients are best treated with short-term crisis intervention, in which the immediate concerns are handled, and symptoms are quickly diminished. Others may require a longer, more intensive form of therapy with the goal of changing behavior or possibly changing character traits. In the former case, the goal is damage control and some restoration of previous equilibrium. In the latter example, a more extensive goal is set, but such therapy tends to have a more permanent solution than short-term intervention.

Although it is not an absolute requirement for practicing psychiatry, most psychiatrists, after completing their training, do take an examination with the American Board of Psychiatry and Neurology and become certified in the field of psychiatry. Many psychiatrists themselves undergo personal psychoanalysis in order to help with their own emotional blind spots and assist them in becoming increasingly sensitive to the therapeutic process.

BASIC ASSUMPTIONS IN PSYCHIATRY

Most practicing psychiatrists accept several basic premises in performing their work. These include at least the following principles: the role of the unconscious, the concept of psychic determinism, the use of defense mechanisms by the ego, the role of transference and countertransference, and the presence of resistance in therapy. These will be discussed in some detail.

It should be mentioned here that these basic assumptions are not the sole province of psychiatry, but are utilized by most psychotherapists regardless of their professional background.

The Role of the Unconscious

Long before Freud postulated the existence of the unconscious in influencing the thoughts, emotions, and behavior of man, others had an idea that forces were present to account for human beings' inconsistency and lack of will. St. Paul, in his memorable statement about the discrepancy between his intentions and his performance, wrote, "The good that I would, I do not, and the evil that I would not, that I do." He spoke of evil forces within himself, warring with his conscience. Both ancient and modern literature deal extensively with these themes.

To my knowledge, Freud was the first one to apply this in a clinical setting. Through his work with hypnosis on patients with hysterical disorders, he discovered that there were indeed other dynamics operating in the mind, which explained the obvious inconsistencies in his patients' feelings and behavior. He theorized that there were powerful forces in the unconscious mind that were not generally known to the conscious mind. Through his clinical cases, he was able to gain access to the unconscious by means of free association (uncensored thoughts; whatever came to mind) and by dreams. He wove this into a treatment tapestry that he called psychoanalysis. Most psychotherapists, with the exception of those who practice only behavioral or cognitive therapy, accept the theory of the unconscious as important in the emotional life of humans.

Psychic Determinism

The principle of psychic determinism was first made clear by Freud in his classic works. It was perhaps best illustrated in his book *The Psychopathology of Everyday Life*, although it is explained in other writings as well.

The basic assumption of this principle is that no mental phenomenon occurs by itself, but that everything has a cause or is at least influenced by causation, even though that cause may be unknown.

One of the tasks of the psychotherapist is to help the patient discover that his actions are not as spontaneous as he might think. Rather, the patient's present actions are based largely on past experience. Most of us do not behave much differently from one day to another. Most individuals function on automatic pilot on a daily basis. When someone acts differently from his expected normal behavior, we are usually surprised. To the extent that a person can take a different view of events and be spontaneous, he allows the possibility for creativity. But, even in creativity there is causality; no act is completely spontaneous.

In the work of psychotherapy, it is common to observe repetitive patterns that patients display. For example, a 38-year-old woman complained about her domineering and overbearing husband. A review of her history revealed that her previous husband had also had these character traits. In fact, she was usually attracted to men who possessed such behavior. She had divorced her first husband because she could not bear his domination. It was not surprising to learn that her father also had the same type of character–charming and engaging, but aggressive and domineering.

Prior to therapy, the patient had no idea that she was attracted to this kind of man based on her past. Freud called this a repetition compulsion; that is, a pattern that tends to repeat itself unless the patient is able to alter his feelings, thoughts, and reactions. Changing these basic patterns is the task of the psychotherapist; it is often difficult to do.

Good therapy might include an alternative to such an approach by helping the patient and her husband understand the nature of the conflict in the marriage, and then working out a compromise. This can be accomplished if there are other strengths to the marriage that make it worthwhile. In the case mentioned here, the patient's husband was able to diminish his aggressiveness sufficiently to satisfy his wife. Simultaneously, she learned to be less sensitive, developed a tougher skin, and learned to confront him with his behavior when he was excessively overbearing. This was accomplished by counseling both husband and wife in joint sessions.

Mechanisms of Defense

The ways in which animals defend themselves are very primitive. They frequently engage in fight or flight reactions when confronted with danger. Our domesticated animals, particularly cats and dogs, are far more subtle and can be observed to illustrate defense mechanisms of the humankind. Withdrawal, acting out, and avoidance are but a few of these defenses.

Defense mechanisms are used to preserve the integrity of the ego or the self. The ego presumably handles conflicts between the id (impulses of sex and aggression) and the superego. The superego consists of both conscious and unconscious aspects. It may be thought of as originating from the sum of all the influences on the individual from her parents, siblings, peer relationships, education, and culture. The superego can sometimes be cruel and punishing. It is the ego's job to use defense mechanisms to arbitrate the needs of the id and superego.

One of the most common defense mechanisms is that of repression. Basically, repression may be viewed as unconscious forgetting. It enables the person to function even when preoccupied with the most serious problems. Perhaps you have had the experience of being totally concerned by a recent tragedy that seems to be on your mind continually. Then, suddenly, you are aware that for the last ten minutes, you have not thought of the tragedy at all. Your mind has repressed the preoccupation and made it possible for you to attend to other activities in your life.

Another mechanism of defense is called sublimation. In this defense, basic drives such as sex or aggression, which may not be appropriate to express in a given time or place, can be diverted to a more socially accepted situation. For example, if you are angry at one of your congregants, you have the option of dealing with your anger directly with her, or your ego can unconsciously deal with your instincts by discharging (sublimating) them by engaging in an active sport.

There are at least a dozen other defense mechanism that are commonly used by us all. They are discussed in more detail in Chapter 7, "The Neuroses."

Transference and Countertransference

In the course of psychotherapy, these two phenomenon are observed frequently. We again have to credit Freud with discovering these transactions. In his analytic work, he became aware of the fact that patients developed feelings toward him that were not easily explainable on the basis of the realty of the situation. Thus, he noted that some of his patients were unduly angry at him, whereas others were in love with him. He postulated the theory that his patients were taking feelings and attitudes from the past and unconsciously placing them into the present therapeutic situation. It became apparent that in psychotherapy, the therapist, at various times, represents the patient's mother, father, or anyone in the past with whom the patient has had a significant relationship. Freud called this transference.

In a similar manner, this phenomenon can occur with the therapist. He also may have feelings and attitudes from the past that he brings into the consultation room without being consciously aware of it. Thus, the therapist may feel overly affectionate or angry toward the patient and not immediately know why. Freud called this countertransference.

Although these concepts were discussed in the previous chapter in regard to the clergyperson and his congregant, they are repeated here in relationship to a clinical setting. To further illustrate these important clinical experiences, the following vignettes are presented. In the course of psychotherapy, these interactions occur constantly.

Transference

A 40-year-old married woman, named Jane, began psychotherapy, with me for symptoms of depression as well as for marital problems. A positive relationship soon developed, and she seemed to relate well. However, one day she appeared very annoyed. I asked her what had happened to cause her to be so upset. At first, she was not aware of any precipitating event to cause her emotional reaction. As I inquired further, she said that she was angry at me, but did not know why. I asked myself what I had said or done to provoke this reaction. Although I could not identify the problem, it gradually became clear to Jane that my manner of speaking and failure to react emotionally to her every word made her angry. She finally said, "You're just like my father. He never paid any attention to me. You men are all alike."

As the therapy progressed, it became apparent that the patient expected men to idolize her and grant her the adoration that her father gave her when she was a child. As she grew up, her father paid less attention to her because he was very involved with his work and he felt very uncomfortable relating to a developing adolescent. The loss that she had experienced with her father was now being transferred onto me in the therapeutic situation. Things from the past were being played out in the present–a typical transference phenomenon.

It was important for Jane to be aware of why she had this reaction during therapy since what occurs in the therapy sessions is a reflection of what goes on in the patient's life. After understanding the transference situation and how Jane expected all men to treat her as her father did when she was a young girl, I turned her attention to her marriage. Was she doing the same thing in her relationship with her husband? Was she expecting him to idolize her at all times? Was he failing to be the adoring male that she cherished in her childhood memories? As we continued therapy, her marriage became more and more the focus of our attention. Although she occasionally became angry at me again, she increasingly recognized the basis for her anger. I repeatedly reminded her that similar periods of anger were probably recurring in her marriage because her husband was not meeting her expectations. Understanding these transference issues was very helpful in dealing with Jane's formerly unrecognized emotional reactions.

At such times in the process of psychotherapy, it is very important for the therapist to understand the historical roots of the patient's emotions. He may choose to acknowledge the feelings of love, hate, anger, or any other emotion that the patient displays toward him without personalizing it. Rather, it is the task of the psychotherapist to inquire into the patient's relationship to parents, siblings, and extended family and explore the emotions engendered in the patient by his family. Only then can one begin to understand the reasons for the exaggerated feelings that occur in the therapy sessions.

In this example, Jane gradually learned how the present therapeutic situation was a repetition of the past relationship with her father. Furthermore, she became aware of her tendency to expect and even demand that men treat her in an adoring manner. Learning about such transference phenomenon can be very beneficial in preventing emotional pain in the future if the patient is able to apply what is learned to her daily life.

Countertransference

In countertransference, the therapist unconsciously takes feelings and attitudes from his past and applies them to the present in the therapeutic process. Something in the patient sets off these emotional reactions in the therapist. This may occur without warning and may be very upsetting to the therapist.

I can recall an example of this phenomenon that occurred when I was working with a married couple. I was in the process of exploring the various difficulties that had been present for the ten years of their marriage. In my previous work with couples, I never had witnessed the extreme anger that these two people were capable of displaying in the therapy sessions. They seemed to care and show love toward each other but were absolutely fierce and unrelenting in their arguments. They also reported that after a violent argument, they could quickly calm down and have a very enjoyable sexual relationship. (This certainly is unusual, but it does happen in some marriages.)

During one of their arguments in a therapy session, the husband turned on me for no apparent reason and let out all his accumulated anger on me. It came as such a surprise that I was alarmed and felt very anxious. He was brutal in his castigation of me. After the first verbal barrage, I am not certain that I heard much more. It literally took my breath away for the moment. I had been in similar situations before with patients who were angry, but I had never reacted in this way. What was different about this reaction? There was something in my background to which I was reacting, but I was not conscious of it at the time. After much reflection on my own past, I became aware of the countertransference aspects going on in this therapeutic relationship. If there was anything that frightened me in my childhood, it was the sudden, seemingly unprovoked wrath of my overworked, irritable father. Although it may not have happened frequently, there were occasions when I became the object of his anger. I might have understood the reason for the angry outbursts if I had been a difficult child. But the anger seemed unrelated to my behavior or at least not in proportion to my transgressions. When my mother chastised me for misbehavior and showed her anger, I had a normal reaction to it. My father's anger petrified me. It was the sudden and unexpected nature of the anger that was difficult for me to handle. This was similar to my patient's unexpected display of anger toward me, and it provoked a similar response. At present, I still do not enjoy unprovoked and unexpected anger directed toward me from others, but I have been able to cope with it in a more normal manner.

It should be noted that transference and countertransference can be positive or negative, depending upon what historically sensitive areas it touches in the unconscious of the patient or therapist. Feelings of love and hate, disappointment and hope, or any other emotion can be elicited in the therapist while he is conducting therapy. It is very important that the therapist understand these phenomena in the course of work with the patients. To do so requires many hours of therapy with patients as well as much supervision, in which these concepts are closely examined. For further comments of this subject, see Chapter 15, "Pastoral Ethics: A Psychiatrist's View."

THE ROLE OF RESISTANCE

There is within all of us, regardless of stated goals and aspirations, the wish to preserve the status quo. Perhaps this is the reason it takes so long to learn new things. Resistance to change can be observed especially in the area of change in behavior and feeling. In psychotherapy, it is difficult to change the patient, even when she is well-motivated. A joke has been made about this: "How many psychiatrists does it take to change a light bulb?" The answer given is, "One, providing the bulb wants to be changed." It generally is easier to change one's thinking process than to alter one's behavior, but it is hardest to change feelings.

The task of the psychotherapist is to overcome the patient's resistance, present the reality of her problems to him or her, and to be an emotional catalyst in the patient's life.

THE COMPETENT PSYCHOTHERAPIST

A fundamental requirement of the therapist is that he or she be a good, dependable listener and capable of trust and empathy. Most patients suffer from injury to self-esteem, partly because of the failure of significant persons in the past to provide for the needs and security that the individuals require. A therapist cannot provide all of these needs, but understanding what they are is essential as a starting point. If a therapist quickly interrupts a patient in the first session to expound on his or her favorite theory, he or she will not be meeting patient's need to ventilate his feelings. The patient will sense the lack of empathy on the therapist's part and be unable to trust him with further details of his life. It may be the patient's first and last session.

Empathy can be recognized by the patient quickly, but trust takes time to develop. I have had some patients tell me very private matters, only after several years of therapy. Some have said to me that it took them years to "trust you with my true feelings."

CHOOSING A PSYCHOTHERAPIST

How does a clergyperson choose a psychotherapist for his or her congregant if asked to do so? Here are some guidelines to follow:

1. Ask your colleagues about the therapists with whom they have worked successfully. In this regard, you would want to know if the therapist has a balanced approach to problems. If he is a psychiatrist, does he use medication when indicated? Does the therapist work cooperatively with the clergy? Does he have a background that can appreciate a patient's religious orientation? I have known of inexperienced therapists who misinterpreted the meaning of religious phrases. For example, if a fundamentalist speaks of God speaking to him or her or hearing the Lord tell him or her to go in a particular direction with life, this could be incorrectly diagnosed by the novice as an auditory hallucination. It is important that a psychotherapist be familiar with the language of various religious groups so that accepted phrases and terms are not confused with psychopathology.

Furthermore, it is important to know if the therapist views religion as a crutch or an unnecessary part of life. Does the therapist feel, just as Karl Marx did, that religion is the "opiate of the people?" Such prejudice could markedly influence the effectiveness of a therapist with a patient who considers religion to be a vital part of life.

2. Another way of evaluating a psychotherapist is to spend a few minutes talking directly with her. It would be quite appropriate to

ask about the therapists' religious background and if she is sensitive to a patient's religious concerns. I do not feel that it is necessary that I have the same religious views as my patients. However, I do think that my own religious training in the Protestant faith and my knowledge of the Bible enable me also to appreciate Catholic and Jewish beliefs in my patients. Incidentally, I do not feel that the psychotherapists' role should include such things as evangelizing, quoting scripture, and engaging in philosophical or religious discussions about her particular beliefs. Such activities should be left to a clergyperson from the particular faith with which the patient is familiar and feels accepted.

A few minutes spent with a psychotherapist will help the clergyperson obtain at least an impression of this individual as a person. Is the therapist arrogant, domineering, passive, hostile, ungiving, or withholding? Does she appear defensive or uncomfortable discussing religious topics? Does she appear empathic and willing to listen to your concerns?

3. Still another way to gauge the appropriateness of a given therapist for your congregant is to call a physician with whom you have a close relationship. Ask him about his referral sources for patients who are in need of psychological or psychiatric care. Most physicians, particularly those in general practice or internal medicine, have a few psychotherapists that they regularly use for consultation or treatment for their patients when needed. Physicians are in a good position to offer information about referrals since they often know therapists personally, socially, and professionally.

When one of my patients moves to another part of the country, to an area where I do not know any psychiatrists, I will tell the patient to ask a friend in the new town to suggest a general practitioner or internist to see there. Consulting with this doctor regarding psychotherapists in the new area usually works well. I find this far superior to looking from someone in a directory of board-qualified psychiatrists or psychologists, although a credentials check might be useful after obtaining a referral.

4. Ultimately, even with careful selection, the patient has to work with a therapist for a while in order to test whether the needs of the patient are met. No amount of screening by the clergyperson is always going to find a successful match. I am sometimes surprised

at the unlikely, or to me, unpredictable relationships that develop between patients and psychotherapists toward an effective treatment. It reminds me of the good friends we have all had, who marry very unlikely mates, and who create unexpectedly good marriages. Nevertheless, some care should be taken to match patient to therapist, whenever this is possible.

5. Perhaps the best recommendation that any psychotherapist could receive is the approval of a patient who has been satisfactorily helped with a particular problem. Success with one patient does not, of course, guarantee success with another, but it does give added confidence to the clergyperson as the referring person.

6. Should the clergy refer a congregant to a social worker, psychologist, psychiatrist, alcohol counselor, or another specialized counselor?

Since I am a psychiatrist, I will confine my remarks to my area of expertise. Psychiatrists are trained in physical medicine and neurology, in addition to obtaining knowledge of mental and emotional diseases. Because of such training, they should be more alert to covert organic problems that may be masquerading as emotional disturbances. Organic disease that is suspected by a psychiatrist may be further diagnosed by an appropriate specialist. If a patient requires medication along with psychotherapy, a psychiatrist, who is properly trained, can provide both. Some psychiatrists have specialized in the use of psychotropic drugs and are called psychopharmacologists. Such physicians do supportive psychotherapy, but depend mostly on medication to control a patient's symptoms.

Other psychiatrists do only psychotherapy and/or psychoanalysis and feel uncomfortable prescribing medications. Such is the case particularly with some older psychiatrists who have been psychoanalytically trained prior to the large-scale introduction of psychotropic drugs. By far, the majority of psychiatrists, however, have been well-trained in psychotherapy and also are quite knowledgeable in the use of medication.

In summary, a psychiatrist should be the first choice as therapist if the following situations exist:

1. The illness is heavily organic in nature or the degree of organicity is questionable.

2. The patient has a schizophrenic disorder, paranoid disorder, or another psychosis of brief duration.
3. The patient has bipolar disorder.
4. Drug abuse or alcoholism and psychosis, severe anxiety, or depression are present concurrently.
5. Severe psychosomatic disorders exist in which hospitalization of the patient is likely to occur. (In such instances, the psychiatrist can usually continue to consult with the patient in the hospital.)

After careful evaluation, some patients in these categories can be transferred to nonpsychiatric psychotherapists. A word of caution: I have seen some clergypersons, who like their fellow counselors in various fields, have rescue fantasies. They have unconscious desires to be the sole helper in their work with their clients. Even when they are clearly working beyond their area of expertise with a very sick person, they continue to operate alone and do not seek outside assistance. Such rescue fantasies cause unnecessary burdens on these counselors, and delay the recovery of and sometimes harm the ailing individual.

Do not be afraid to ask for help! It is no reflection on your ability. Rather, it is a sign of maturity to know when to seek the proper consultation. Save your energies for areas in which you can be more effective.

Chapter 17

Conclusion

The clergy are constantly on the front line in life and death matters. They may be the first to see the pain of the physically and emotionally ill, the first to be consulted by disturbed relatives when family disruptions occur, and the first to support the grieving family when a death occurs. The clergy carry a necessary but heavy burden in conducting the care of their congregants.

Given the difficult task that each clergyperson has in working with a congregation, he or she needs all the help from God and others that can be obtained. This includes a good education, a continuing interest in his or her emotional development and growth, a supportive family, and supportive colleagues. The clergyperson also needs to know as much as possible about how to best assist his or her congregants to help themselves in their own growth toward mental and spiritual maturity.

Why should the clergy be informed about mental and emotional illnesses? Why is such information important to the clergy? There are a number of reasons, all of which I have alluded to in the chapters of this book.

In their role as counselors, the clergy can be very helpful in recognizing various psychological problems and assisting their congregants with such difficulties or guiding them to the proper sources of help. The clergy often have close, trusting relationships with their congregants, which exceed those of many family members and friends. If a clergyperson makes a recommendation to a congregant, it may be more quickly followed than when the same advice comes from someone else. If the clergyperson is not familiar with the help that is available to him or her from the mental health field, he or she may be working toward conflicting goals with a psychotherapist and not even be aware of it. It is very important in some cases that the clergyperson and the psychotherapist communicate about a person who they have as their common concern. Furthermore, by being better informed about what is available, the clergy can be of help obtaining faster treatment of organic illnesses, severe depression, and psychoses, all of which require psychiatric treatment.

It is important that the clergyperson know the difference between true guilt, neurotic guilt, and guilt that is of a psychotic nature. The latter is not the type that can be treated by pastoral counseling or the psychotherapist, who is not a psychiatrist, because hospitalization and medication may be necessary for effective treatment.

With a knowledge of personality disorders, the clergyperson can recognize the strengths and weaknesses in his or her congregants. By so doing, he or she can better utilize each congregant in the service of the congregation without the frustration of having the congregant working in an unsuitable job because of particular personality traits.

An awareness of the phenomena of transference and countertransference can be of great help to the clergyperson because it can assist him or her in understanding congregants' unexpected and unusual emotional responses or his or her own unanticipated emotional reactions. Without such knowledge, a clergyperson can become unnecessarily involved with congregants in very disruptive emotional relationships.

To the extent possible, the clergyperson should take care of his or her own needs so that he or she is emotionally stable and has the energy to undertake the difficult task of working with congregants. Too much commitment is as bad as not enough. "All work and no play" applies to the clergy as well as to anyone else.

Our mutual goal should be to have each person–congregant or patient–live as full a life as possible, helping each to reach his or her greatest potential for physical, cognitive, and spiritual development. To the degree that we in our respective professions can accomplish this goal, we also fulfill our own needs for growth.

In essence, we are all healers of the soul–psychotherapists by the analysis of mental dynamics, and the clergy through ritual, theology, and inspiration. We in our various professions need each other.

The human mind and soul are too complicated to be helped in only one way.

The clergy have been with us since the early history of humankind. Psychotherapy, as a specific method of counseling, has been a recent phenomenon used to assist persons with mental and emotional problems. It was made possible by economic and social changes that have occurred with the growth of civilization. Today, when a congregant has the need for psychotherapy and is able to find a good working relationship with a therapist while also enjoying the spiritual nourishment afforded by the clergy, that person is twice blessed.

It is my firm conviction that psychotherapists of all kinds should become more apprised of the importance of religious influences on the lives of their patients, and that the clergy should be well-informed about mental illness and what is available to them from the field of mental health. Only with such knowledge can the clergy be fully aware of how they can participate in assisting congregants; they also must know when and to whom to refer congregants for psychotherapeutic counseling.

Not until recently did I become consciously aware of why I began writing this book. It occurred to me that I could have used an informed clergyperson during my adolescence to advise me on personal matters and possibly to refer me for counseling to a psychotherapist. When I was 16 years old, my father died unexpectedly. He was 65 years of age. We were a lower-middle-class immigrant Dutch family. I had never had a ten-minute conversation with my father that I could remember. Some of my brothers were old enough to be my father. They tried to father me as best they could in the limited time that was available to them, but no one ever addressed the lack of relationship between my father and me, nor the grieving that should have been done in regard to my father's death. Perhaps everyone was addressing their own grief. Only recently did this awareness become a reality and a concern when I read the book *Iron John* by Robert Bly. In this insightful book, the author makes some basic observations about men from fairy tales, mythology, and religion. Among these, he speaks of a man's need to relate to his father in life and to properly mourn his father's death.

There was little positive relationship with my father while he was alive, and there was no one around me to assist in mourning my father's death. The clergyperson, who was present at the time, stands out in my memory as being more concerned with our heinous sin, to which he referred frequently, than to the emotional and spiritual needs of his young congregants. He left me to fend for myself, and I later left that congregation to be received more warmly by a pastor who was more concerned with the richness and joy of the spiritual journey than with heinous sin.

This book is written with the hope that the members of the clergy who read these pages will help to make their congregants' lives a little less difficult at the time when they most need the comfort and support that is required for life's difficult moments. I wish that I had been able to talk with my father about life, about his experience in the Netherlands, about why he had to emigrate with his large family, about how he managed to work for a year to raise enough money to bring his family to the United States, about the difficulty of being unemployed during the Depression, and many other things that I will never know. Perhaps then I would have been able to mourn in a meaningful way. It is a relationship that is incomplete—one that will never be finished.

In our present secular society, the clergy is little recognized, even though they do much to help their congregants with difficult emotional and spiritual concerns. Society needs the clergy more than most people know.

Bibliography

General

Frances A, Pincus HA, First MB, et al. *Diagnostic and statistical manual of mental disorders*, 4th ed. Washington, DC: American Psychiatric Press, 1994.

Kaplan HI, Sadock BJ (eds.). *Comprehensive textbook of psychiatry*, 6th ed. Volumes 1 and 2. Baltimore: Williams & Wilkins, 1994.

Kaplan HI, Sadock BJ, and Grebb JA. *Synopsis of psychiatry*, 7th ed. Baltimore: Williams & Wilkins, 1994.

Goldman, HH. *Review of general psychiatry*, 2nd ed. Englewood Cliffs, NJ: Appleton and Lange, Prentice Hall, 1988.

Stoudmire A. *Human behavior*, 2nd ed. Philadelphia: J.B. Lippincott, 1994.

Stoudmire A. *Clinical psychiatry*, 2nd ed. Philadelphia: J.B. Lippincott, 1994.

Talbott J, Hales RE, Yudofsky S (eds.). *Textbook of psychiatry*, 2nd ed. Washington, DC: American Psychiatric Press, 1994.

Chapter 1

Cousins N. *Head first*. New York: E.P. Dutton, 1989.

Fromm E. *Psychoanalysis and religion*. New Haven, CT: Yale University Press, 1950.

Freud S. *Future of an illusion*. New York: Norton, 1975.

Peale NV. *The power of positive thinking*. New York: Ballantine, 1990.

Chapter 2

Freud S. *Complete psychological works of Sigmund Freud*. London: Hogarth Press, 1953-1966.

Golden LR, Gershon ES. Association and linkage studies of genetic marker loci in major psychiatric disorders. *Psychiatric Dev* 4: 387-418, 1983.

Rainer JD. Genetics and psychiatry. In: Kaplan HI, Sadock BJ (eds.). *Comprehensive textbook of psychiatry*, 5th ed. Baltimore: Williams & Wilkins, 1989.

Schuckit MA. Genetic and clinical implications of alcoholism and affective disorders. *American J Psychiatry* 143:140, 1986.

Chapter 3

Judd LL, Groves PM. *Psychobiological foundations of clinical psychiatry.* Philadelphia: J.B. Lippincott, 1986.

Szasz T. *The myth of mental illness.* New York: Hoeber, 1962.

Chapter 4

Kaplan HI, Sadock BJ. Mood disorders (pp. 516-572). In: *Synopsis of psychiatry.* Baltimore: Williams & Wilkins, 1988.

Klerman GL. History and developments of modern concepts of affective illness. In, Post RM, Ballenger JC (ed.). *Neurobiology of mood disorders*, 1-19. Baltimore: Williams & Wilkins, 1984.

Chapter 5

Arieti S. *Interpretation of schizophrenia*, 2nd ed. New York: Basic Books, 1974.

Green H. *I never promised you a rose garden.* New York: Signet, 1964.

Kaplan B. *The inner world of mental illness.* New York: Harper & Row, 1964.

Low AA. *Mental health through will training.* North Quincy, MA: Christopher Publishing, 1950.

Scheider K. *Clinical psychopathology.* New York: Grune & Stratton, 1959.

Sullivan HS. *Schizophrenia as a human process.* New York: Norton, 1962.

Chapter 6: Refer to General References

Chapter 7

Freud A. *The ego and the mechanisms of defense.* New York: International University Press, 1946.

Griest JH, Jefferson JW. *Anxiety and its treatment: Help is available.* Washington, DC: American Psychiatric Press, 1986.

Horney K. *The neurotic personality of our times.* Norton, 1947.

Schriber FR. *Sybil.* New York: Warner Paperback, 1973.

Thigpen CH, Thigpen H, Cleckley HM. *The three faces of Eve.* New York: McGraw-Hill, 1957.

Chapter 8

Schuckit MA. *Drug and alcohol abuse. A clinical guide to diagnosis and treatment.* New York: Plenum Press, 1979.

Smith DE, Gay DR (eds.). *It's so good, don't even try it once.* New York: Prentice Hall, 1972.

Beattie M. *Codependent no more.* San Francisco: Harper & Row, 1987.

Chapter 9

Lishman WA. *Organic psychiatry*, 2nd ed. New York: Oxford, Blackwell Scientific Publication, 1987.

Yesavage J. Dementia: Differential diagnosis and treatment. *Geriatrics* 34:51-59, 1979.

Yudofsky SC, Hales RD (eds.). *Textbook of neuropsychiatry*, 2nd ed. Washington, DC: American Psychiatric Press, 1992.

Chapter 10

Cooper AM, Frances AJ, Sacks MH, et al. *The personality disorders and neuroses.* Philadelphia: J.B. Lippincott, 1986.

Kernberg O. *Borderline conditions and pathological narcissism.* New York: Jason Aronson, 1975.

Thomas A, Chess S. *Temperament and development.* New York: Brunner/Mazel, 1977.

Chapter 11

Bolby J. *Attachment and loss*, Volume 3. *Loss, sadness, and depression.* New York: Basic Books, 1980.

Freud S. *Mourning and melancholia* (1917). In: *Standard edition of the complete psychological works of Sigmund Freud*, Volume 14. London: Hogarth Press, 1957.

James J, Cherry F. *The grief recovery handbook.* New York: Harper-Collins, 1989.

Kübler-Ross E. *On death and dying.* New York: Macmillan, 1969.

Chapter 12

Kaplan HS. *The new sex therapy.* New York: Brunner/Mazel, 1974.

Kaplan HS. *Sexual aversion, sexual phobias, and panic disorders.* New York: Brunner/Mazel, 1987.

Kaplan L. *The temptations of Emma Bovary.* New York: Doubleday, 1991.

Kinsey AC. *Sexual behavior in the human male.* Philadelphia: W.B. Saunders, 1948.

Masters WH, Johnson VE. *Human sexual response.* Boston: Little Brown, 1966.

Masters WH, Johnson VE. *Human sexual inadequacy.* Boston: Little Brown, 1970.

Chapter 13

Agras WS. *Eating disorders: Management of obesity, bulimia, and anorexia nervosa.* Oxford, NY: University Press, 1987.

Bruch H. *Eating disorders: Obesity, anorexia, and the person within.* New York: Basic Books, 1973.

Zraly K, Swoft D. *Anorexia, bulimia, and compulsive overeating.* New York: Continuum, 1990.

Chapter 14

Benson H. *The relaxation response.* New York: William Morrow, 1976.

Gawain S. *Creative visualization.* New York: Bantam, 1985.

Hanson PG. *The joy of stress*. Kansas City, KA: Andrews and McMeel, 1986.

Levinson DJ. *The seasons of a man's life*. New York: Ballantine, 1978.

Selye H. *Stress without distress*. New York: New American Library, 1974.

Sheehy G. *Passages*. New York: Bantam, 1984.

Sullivan HS. *Conceptions of modern psychiatry*. Norton, 1947.

Tennyson AL. *Idylls of the King*. New York: New American Library of World Literature, p. 251, 1961.

Chapter 15

Freud A. *The ego and the mechanisms of defense*. New York: International University Press, 1946.

Chapter 16

Freud S. *The psychopathology of everyday life*, In: Standard edition of the complete psychological works of Sigmund Freud. London: Hogarth Press, 1955.

Index